Healthcare Simulation Education

Healthcare Simulation Education

Healthcare Simulation Education

Evidence, Theory and Practice

EDITED BY

Debra Nestel
The University of Melbourne & Monash University, Victoria, Australia

Michelle Kelly
Curtin University, Western Australia, Australia

Brian Jolly
University of Newcastle, New South Wales, Australia

Marcus Watson
University of Queensland, Queensland, Australia

WILEY Blackwell

Section VI: Conclusions and future practice

Contributors

Pamela B. Andreatta PhD EdD CHSE
Institute for Simulation and Training, University of
Central Florida College of Medicine, Orlando, FL, USA

Rafidah Atan MBBS MAnaes FANZCA EDIC GradCert-
ClinSim GradCertHigherEd
Monash University Malaysia, Johor Bahru, Malaysia

Komal Bajaj MD MHPEd
New York City Health & Hospitals, New York, USA

Margaret Bearman PhD BComp (Hons) Cert PA
Centre for Research and Assessment in Digital Learning
(CRADLE), Deakin University, Victoria, Australia

Adam Cheng MD FRCPC
Section of Emergency Medicine, Alberta Children's
Hospital, Calgary, Canada
Department of Paediatrics, University of Calgary,
Calgary, Canada

Ian Civil CNZM MBE (Mil) KStJ ED MBChB FRACS
FACS
Faculty of Medical and Health Sciences, University of
Auckland, Auckland, New Zealand

Teresa Crea DCA
University of Canberra – Centre for Creative and
Cultural Research, Canberra, Australia
Asia Pacific Simulation Alliance, South Australia &
Australian Capital Territory, Australia

Dick Davies
Ambient Performance Ltd, London

Parvati Dev PhD
Los Altos Hills, California, USA

Chaoyan Dong PhD MS CHSE
Sengkang Health, Singapore

Mike Eddie BMBS BMedSci (Hons)
Dorset County Hospital, Dorchester, United Kingdom

Simon Edgar MBChB FRCA MScEd FAcadMEd
NHS Lothian, Edinburgh, Scotland

Nathan Emmerich PhD
School of History, Anthropology, Politics and Philosophy
Queen's University Belfast, Northern Ireland, UK

Walter Eppich MD MEd
Departments of Pediatrics and Medical Education,
Northwestern University Feinberg School of Medicine,
Illinois, USA

Mick Fielding BEng PhD
Institute for Intelligent Systems Research and Innovation (IISRI), Deakin University, Australia

Kirsty J. Freeman BNurs PGradDipMid GradDipEd
CHSE
WA Country Health Service, Perth, Australia

Jonathan Gatward BSc MBChB FRCA DICM FCICM
Cert Ed FHEA
Intensive Care Unit, Royal North Shore Hospital, St
Leonards, Australia
University of Sydney, Sydney, Australia

Gerard Gormley MD FRCGP FHEA
School of Medicine, Dentistry and Biomedical Sciences,
Centre for Medical Education, Queen's University
Belfast, Northern Ireland
The Wilson Centre, University of Toronto, Faculty of
Medicine and University Health Network, Toronto,
Canada

Suzanne Gough BSc (Hons) MA Ed (Research) PhD
PGC-AP Physiotherapy PFHEA
Department of Health Professions, Manchester
Metropolitan University, Manchester, UK

Vincent Grant MD FRCPC
Departments of Paediatrics and Emergency Medicine,
Cumming School of Medicine, University of Calgary,
Calgary, Canada

Stephen Guinea PhD
Faculty of Health Sciences, Australian Catholic University, Victoria, Australia

Carrie Hamilton RGN BSc MSc
Training and Innovation, SimComm Academy, Southampton, UK

Owen Hammett BN DipIMC (RCSEd) RN
University Hospital Southampton NHS Foundation Trust, Southampton, UK

Fei Han MD PhD
Tianjin Medical University, Tianjin, China

William L. Heinrichs MD PhD
Stanford University, California, USA

LY Ho MBBS MRCS FCSHK FHKAM(Surgery) FRCSEd(Urol)
Queen Elizabeth Hospital, Hospital Authority, Hong Kong SAR

Phil Hyde BSc BM MRCPCH FRACP FFICM FIMC RCSEd
Southampton Children's Hospital, Southampton, UK
Dorset and Somerset Air Ambulance, Wellington, UK

Brian Jolly BSc(Hons) MA(Ed) PhD
School of Medicine & Public Health, Faculty of Health and Medicine, University of Newcastle, New South Wales, Australia

Michelle Kelly PhD MN BSc RN
Curtin University, Perth, Australia

Bee Leng Sabrina Koh RN MHSc(Ed) PGDip(CC) BN CHSE
Sengkang Health, Singapore

Michaela Kolbe PhD PD
University Hospital Zurich, Simulation Center, Zurich, Switzerland

Kristian Krogh MD PhD
Department of Anaesthesia and Intensive Care, Aarhus University Hospital, Aarhus, Denmark
Centre for Health Sciences Education, Aarhus University, Aarhus, Denmark

Arunaz Kumar MBBS MD MRCOG FRANZCOG GCHPE
Faculty of Medicine Nursing and Allied Health, Monash University, Clayton, Australia
Department of Obstetrics and Gynaecology, Monash Health, Clayton, Australia

Hani Lababidi MD FCCP
Center for Research, Education & Simulation Enhanced Training (CRESENT), King Fahad Medical City, Riyadh, Saudi Arabia

Ralph J. MacKinnon BSc MBChB FRCA
Department of Paediatric Anaesthesia, Royal Manchester Children's Hospital, Manchester, UK

Kenny Macleod MScOR
TMN Simulation, Melbourne, Australia

Stuart Marshall MBChB MHumanFact MRCA FANZCA
Department of Anaesthesia and Perioperative Medicine, Monash University, Victoria, Australia

Alistair May BSc MBBS FRCA
Scottish Centre for Simulation and Clinical Human Factors, Forth Valley Royal Hospital, Larbert, Scotland

Melissa McCullough PhD FHEA
School of Medicine, Department of Clinical Medicine, Brighton & Sussex Medical School, Brighton, UK

Cate McIntosh MBBS FANZCA
Hunter New England Simulation Centre, John Hunter Hospital, Newcastle, Australia

Leigh McKay RN BAS (Nursing) MPH Cert Intensive Care
NSW Organ & Tissue Donation Service, Kogarah, Australia

Nancy McNaughton MEd PhD
Centre for Learning Innovation and Simulation, Michener Institute of Education, Wilson Centre for Research in Education, University Health Network, Toronto, Canada

Michael Meguerdichian MD MHPEd
New York City Health & Hospitals, New York, USA

Michael Moneypenny BSc(Hons) MBChB(Hons) MD FRCA FHEA
Scottish Centre for Simulation and Clinical Human Factors, Forth Valley Royal Hospital, Larbert, Scotland

Robert Moody
St. Vincents Hospital, Melbourne, Australia

Saeid Nahavandi BSc (Hons) MSc PhD
Institute for Intelligent Systems Research and Innovation (IISRI), Deakin University, Australia

Zoran Najdovski BEng PhD
Institute for Intelligent Systems Research and Innovation (IISRI), Deakin University, Australia

Debra Nestel PhD FAcadMEd CHSE-A
Department of Surgery, Melbourne Medical School, Melbourne, Australia
Faculty of Medicine, Dentistry & Health Sciences, University of Melbourne, Melbourne, Australia
Faculty of Medicine, Nursing & Health Sciences, Monash University, Victoria, Australia

George Ng MBBS MRCP FHKCP FHKAM(Medicine) FCICM MPH
Queen Elizabeth Hospital, Hospital Authority, Hong Kong SAR

Harry Owen MB BCh MD FANZCA
School of Medicine, Flinders University, Adelaide, Australia

Richard Page BMedSci MBBS FRACS (Orth) FAOrthA
School of Medicine, Faculty of Health, Deakin University, Australia

Naganathan MBBS FRCPI AM
Monash University Malaysia, Johor Bahru, Johor

Jessica Pohlman MPA MEd
New York City Health & Hospitals, New York, USA

Kate Pryde BMedSci BMBS MRCPCH
Southampton Children's Hospital, Southampton, UK

Jill Sanko PhD MS ARNP CHSE-A
University of Miami, School of Nursing and Health Studies, Coral Gables, FL, USA

Taylor Sawyer DO MEd CHSE-A
Seattle Children's Hospital, Seattle, WA, USA

Eric So MBBS FHKCA FHKAM(Anaesthesiology) BSc (Biomedical Science) PGDipEcho
Queen Elizabeth Hospital, Hospital Authority, Hong Kong SAR

Suneet Sood MBBS MS MAMS
Monash University Malaysia, Johor Bahru, Malaysia

Kim Sykes MBChB DCH MRCPCH FFICM
Southampton Children's Hospital, Southampton, UK

Katie Walker RN MBA
New York City Health & Hospitals, New York, USA

Marcus Watson PhD
School of Medicine and School of Psychology, University of Queensland, Queensland, Australia

Matthew Watson BEng PhD
Institute for Intelligent Systems Research and Innovation (IISRI), Deakin University, Australia

Lei Wei BEng PhD
Institute for Intelligent Systems Research and Innovation (IISRI), Deakin University, Australia

Jenny Weller MD MClinEd MBBS FANZCA FRCA
Centre for Medical and Health Sciences Education, University of Auckland, Auckland, New Zealand
Auckland City Hospital, Auckland, New Zealand

Nor'azim Mohd Yunos MBBS MAnaes EDIC GradCertHigherEd
Monash University Malaysia, Johor Bahru, Malaysia

Hailing Zhou BEng PhD
Institute for Intelligent Systems Research and Innovation (IISRI), Deakin University, Australia

Acknowledgements

We acknowledge the contributions of the following colleagues:

Fernando Bello, Peter Brooks, Roberta Brown, Chris Browne, Dylan Campher, Chris Christophi, John Collins, Jane Dacre, Stephen Duckett, Rosalind Elliott, Richard Fielding, Brendan Flanagan, Carol Goldstein, Carolyn Hayes, Robert Herkes, Jane Kidd, Roger Kneebone, Ellie McCann, Liz Molloy, NSW Organ and Tissue Donation Service, Stephanie O'Regan, Lin Perry, Julie Potter, Ray Raper, Adam Roshan, Peter Saul, Myra Sgorbini, Patsy Stark, Robyn Tamblyn, UTS: Health Laboratory Staff, UTS: Health Simulation Technicians, Leonie Watterson and Christopher Williams.

In memory of Adelle Collins, who provided project support to form the Australian Society for Simulation in Healthcare.

Debra Nestel, Michelle Kelly, Brian Jolly, Marcus Watson

SECTION I
Introduction

CHAPTER 1

An introduction to healthcare simulation

Debra Nestel & Michelle Kelly

KEY MESSAGES

- Healthcare simulation plays a critical role in patient safety.
- There are benefits of integrating simulation in all phases of education and training of individuals involved in the provision of healthcare.
- Although simulation modalities are diverse, there appear to be commonalities in designing for learning using simulation.
- The focus of this book is on simulation as an educational method.

Overview

This chapter introduces essential concepts for simulation-based education (SBE) in healthcare. The role of patient safety as an endpoint for many healthcare simulation practices is highlighted. The chapter also orientates readers to the book. There are six sections, this chapter being the first, the second on theoretical perspectives and frameworks, the third on contemporary issues, the fourth on elements of simulation practice, the fifth on innovations in simulation and, finally, the sixth, crystal ball gazing 20 years from now. We invite readers to work through the book sequentially. However, it is also designed so that each section and chapter can be reviewed independently.

Introduction

Simulation offers an important route to safer care for patients and needs to be more fully integrated into the health service.
Sir Liam Donaldson (2009)

In 2009, the Chief Medical Officer in the United Kingdom, Sir Liam Donaldson, wrote that *simulation* was one of the top priorities of the health services for the next decade [1]. He emphasized the role of simulation in rehearsal for emergency situations, for the development of teamwork and for learning psychomotor skills in settings and at times that do not place patients at risk. He also questioned the logic of charging clinicians to undertake training to make their practice safer. Although progress has been made in some areas, much remains to be done. In this book we share some of these advances, offer guidance in others and explore new ideas and practices.

Professor David Gaba, a pioneer in healthcare simulation, is widely quoted for the following definition: 'Simulation is a technique – not a technology – to replace or amplify real experiences with guided experiences that evoke or replicate substantial aspects of the real world in a fully interactive manner' [2]. This definition sits well in the educational context for which it was developed. Like Donaldson, Gaba argues for integrated training approaches where 'clinical personnel, teams, and systems should undergo continual systematic training, rehearsal, performance assessment and refinement in their practice' [2].

Most healthcare simulation has patient safety as its ultimate goal. The drivers for SBE are well reported and include the expanding numbers of health professional students and clinicians balanced with constraints on work time. There is a shift to competency-based education and growing evidence supporting SBE as a strategic instructional approach [3, 4]. Healthcare simulation has a long history that includes images, layered transparencies, tactile models and simulated (standardized) patients [5–7]. Developments in computer-driven technologies such as task trainers, mannequin simulators

Healthcare Simulation Education: Evidence, Theory and Practice, First Edition.
Edited by Debra Nestel, Michelle Kelly, Brian Jolly and Marcus Watson.
© 2018 John Wiley & Sons Ltd. Published 2018 by John Wiley & Sons Ltd.

share experiences of using simulation to enhance safe practices of home birthing in Australia (Chapter 22); Gough describes her experiences of video-reflexivity to amplify learning through simulations (Chapter 23); and Gatward et al. document the outcomes of SBE to augment the national organ and tissue donation requestor training programme (Chapter 24).

At the meso level, from a curriculum perspective, Han writes about his journey in reconfiguring and integrating SBE into a medical degree in China (Chapter 25). Next, Atan et al. provide their collective experience of using simulation to help junior doctors identify critical elements of transporting critically ill patients in Malaysia (Chapter 26). Koh and Dong share their success in creating a programme to extend the role of simulation technicians (Chapter 27). This initiative in Singapore and Malaysia has led to increased job satisfaction and retention and continuity of simulation centre operations.

Finally, we feature four macro-level initiatives that focus on the organizational or systems level of healthcare practice and delivery. Labibidi offers insights into the challenges of planning simulation for a unique healthcare facility in Saudi Arabia – the King Fahad Medical City – comprising four hospitals, four specialized medical centres and a Faculty of Medicine (Chapter 28). An integrated approach to simulation was adopted through central governance and funding, which still allows a level of independence in educational content and delivery in separate facilities. So and Ng write about the importance and benefits of establishing partnerships early in the process of developing a new simulation centre (Chapter 29). The example, from Hong Kong, highlights a tripartite relationship with leaders from the simulation centre, the hospital and the broader health authority. The impact of simulation on groups and their interactions is illustrated by Eddie et al., who report on the benefits of testing workflow and patient care processes in a new paediatric emergency department (Chapter 30). And finally, from Macleod and Moody comes a case study from simulation modelling showing how the configuration of space design features can be manipulated to maximize work efficiencies and patient flow (Chapter 31). In summary, these innovations illustrate the diversity of the application of simulation in healthcare contexts.

In the final section we look to the future of healthcare simulation. Crystal ball gazing, we consider directions for practice drawing on the contents of this book and our own experiences. We are enormously grateful to our colleagues for sharing their expertise in healthcare simulation to advance our practices.

References

1 Donaldson, L. (2009) *150 years of the Chief Medical Officer's Annual Report 2008*, Department of Health, London.

2 Gaba, D. (2007) The future vision of simulation in healthcare. *Simul Healthc.*, **2**, 126–35.

3 Bearman, M., Nestel, D. and Andreatta, P. (2013) Simulation-based medical education, in *The Oxford book of medical education* (ed. K. Walsh), Oxford University Press, Oxford, pp. 186–97.

4 Nestel, D., Watson, M., Bearman, M. *et al.* (2013) Strategic approaches to simulation-based education: a case study from Australia. *J Health Spec*, **1** (1), 4–12.

5 Owen, H. (2012) Early use of simulation in medical education. *Simul Healthc*, **7** (2), 102–16.

6 Bradley, P. (2006) The history of simulation in medical education and possible future directions. *Med Educ*, **40** (3), 254–62. doi: 10.1111/j.1365-2929.2006.02394.x

7 Howley L, Gliva-McConvey G, Thornton J. Standardized patient practices: initial report on the survey of US and Canadian medical schools. *Med Educ Online.* 2009;**14**(7), 127. doi: 10.3885/meo.2009.F0000208

8 Nestel, D., Bearman, M., Brooks, P. *et al.* (2016) A national training program for simulation educators and technicians: evaluation strategy and outcomes. *BMC Med Educ.*, **16**, 25. doi: 10.1186/s12909-016-0548-x

9 Navedo, D. and Simon, R. (2013) Specialized courses in simulation, in *The comprehensive textbook of healthcare simulation* (eds A. Levine, S. DeMaria, A. Schwartz and A. Sim), Springer, New York, pp. 593–7.

10 Watson, K., Wright, A., Morris, N. *et al.* (2012) Can simulation replace part of clinical time? Two parallel randomised controlled trials. *Med Educ*, **46** (7), 657–67. doi: 10.1111/j.1365-2923.2012.04295.x

11 Hayden, J., Smily, R., Alexander, M. *et al.* (2014) The NCSBN National Simulation Study: a longitudinal, randomized, controlled study replacing clinical hours with simulation in prelicensure nursing education. *J Nurs Regul*, **5** (2 Supplement), S1–S64.

12 Rosenthal, M., Ritter, E., Goova, M. *et al.* (2010) Proficiency-based fundamentals of laparoscopic surgery skills training results in durable performance improvement and a uniform certification pass rate. *Surg Endosc.*, **10**, 2453–7. doi: 10.1007/s00464-010-0985-2

13 Simulation Australasia. SimHealth conference [cited 2 February 2016]. Available from: http://www.simulationaustralasia.com/events/simhealth

14 Arora S, Sevdalis N. HOSPEX and concepts of simulation. *J R Army Med Corps.* 2008;**154**(3):202–5. PubMed PMID: 19202831.

SECTION II
Theoretical perspectives and frameworks for healthcare simulation

CHAPTER 2

Theories informing healthcare simulation practice

Margaret Bearman, Debra Nestel & Nancy McNaughton

KEY MESSAGES

- Learning theories are guides rather than prescriptions.
- Learning theories align with different ways of understanding the nature of knowledge.
- Behaviourism emphasizes the achievement of an external standard through demonstrated behaviours; elements of 'deliberate practice' reflect behaviourist principles.
- Constructivism is a broad umbrella term for theories concerned with individual and social constructions of knowledge, many with great relevance to simulation-based education.
- Critical theory approaches focus outward on society and its effect on simulation practices.

Overview

Theories can be considered coherent frameworks of ideas, which inform learning and other simulation practices. This chapter provides a brief overview of different types of theories, illustrated by selected theorists and examples of application to practice. The first section provides a short overview of behaviourism and some of the key debates, as well as expanding on an additional theory, *deliberate practice*, which draws from behaviourist principles. The next section starts by describing constructivist approaches associated with theories such as *reflective practice*, before going on to explore a social learning theory, *situated learning*. The final section articulates the broad premise of critical theories, before focusing on one theorist, *Michel Foucault*, and providing an exploration of simulated

patient (SP) practice through a critical theory lens. The development of patient-focused simulation is presented as an example of how theory can be applied to develop simulation practice.

Introduction

Ideas about how people learn underpin simulation-based education (SBE) in the health professions. When these ideas are formalized into coherent frameworks, they are referred to as *learning theories*. Learning theories permit educators to identify teaching approaches that can optimize the opportunity afforded by the simulation encounter, and thereby assist learners to acquire new knowledge or skills. They can be purely conceptual or derived from the rigorous collection of qualitative and quantitative data. Learning theories are not absolute; they guide rather than prescribe. Educators draw on them for different reasons. For example, theories can support the initial educational design such as making decisions about what simulation method to choose and why; they can assist with resolving specific dilemmas such as how to manage underperforming learners; or they can challenge accepted practices such as a longstanding approach to debriefing.

This overview of theories that inform healthcare simulation practice can assist in guiding simulation design, development, implementation and facilitation. It is by no means comprehensive, but gives an indication of both the value and the diversity of theories informing SBE. We provide our perspectives as SBE practitioners, researchers and scholars, noting that this is an area in which there is no definite expert consensus.

Healthcare Simulation Education: Evidence, Theory and Practice, First Edition.
Edited by Debra Nestel, Michelle Kelly, Brian Jolly and Marcus Watson.
© 2018 John Wiley & Sons Ltd. Published 2018 by John Wiley & Sons Ltd.

Learning theories are often very abstract. Educators may find theory most helpful by considering its value within local professional and environmental contexts. For example, the legacy of Western political domination may seem irrelevant to SBE, but thinking about this in theoretical terms can prompt educators to review whether their simulators and SP represent the skin colour and physical appearance of the local community.

We suggest that learning theories can be aligned with ways of understanding knowledge (epistemology) and reality (ontology). This chapter presents three overlapping categories of learning theories, which align with particular notions of knowledge and reality. *Behaviourist* learning theories align most easily with worldviews that are concerned with objective truths and measurement. These theories are less concerned with the internal mechanisms of learners, and more with their behaviours, which can be observed. *Constructivist* theories are focused on the learner's role in learning, while *social learning* theories extend this to consider the role of the learning environment. Both of these approaches are concordant with a worldview that is concerned with individual and social constructions of knowledge. Finally, *critical theories* consider the broader questions of society and social behaviours. These are not learning theories per se, but provide valuable lessons on understanding how the broader sociocultural context may influence learning. It is worth noting that there is little consensus on the categorization of learning theories and that educators draw from multiple theories for diverse reasons. We will present some of this complexity in our discussion while maintaining the focus on the practical value of learning theories to SBE.

Behaviourism

Behaviourism, unlike the other categories in this chapter, can be considered a coherent theory as well as a pedagogy. Behaviourism's dominance of the educational literature has waxed and waned over the last 80 years. Its current place in the learning theory landscape is controversial. Some people consider it to be primarily a notion of learning as response to a stimulus, and certainly Ivan Pavlov, a notable historical influence, studied stimulus and response in animals [1]. Rote learning, such as memorizing the sum '7 × 8 = 56', is a simple example of this. In this instance, '7 × 8' is the

stimulus and '56' is the learnt response. Behaviourism was once seen as being superseded by a cognitive view of learning [2], but over time discourses about behaviourism have continued to develop. Those who draw on it today distinguish a range of more nuanced features, although they still hold to the basic premise of stimulus and response [1].

We broadly define contemporary behaviourism as those approaches to learning that focus on achieving an external standard that must be achieved through demonstrated behaviours. This aligns with Woollard's view [1] that 'behaviourism, in terms of learning, considers that it is through modifying behaviour and ensuring learners' preparedness for learning that the best outcomes will be achieved. Behaviourism embraces a pedagogy built upon precision, rigour, analysis, measurement and outcomes' (p. 22). These notions provide the foundation for many of our historical educational practices. For example, the writing of learning objectives focuses on demonstrable change in behaviours, as proposed by Ralph Tyler in 1949 [3]. Equally, accreditation of learning with its concerns about valid and reliable assessment also aligns with behaviourist principles.

There are some areas where we think behaviourism is most valuable in SBE. In particular, health professional practice is full of simple and complex practices, which should occur automatically without the practitioner thinking deeply about how to complete the tasks as they do them. These activities can be psychomotor skills such as suturing, cognitive tasks such as pattern recognition, or even communication skills, such as always introducing oneself to the patient or healthcare consumer by name. These activities are also often well taught in simulation, due to the emphasis on repetitive practice to ensure automaticity.

McGaghie et al. [4], in their 2011 critical review, noted a number of 'best practices' in SBE that draw from behaviourist principles. One of these is *deliberate practice*, which is presented as an example of a theory with particular relevance to SBE. *Deliberate practice* was conceptualized by Anders Ericsson, a cognitive psychologist, who sought to understand how elite performers achieved excellence [5]. From this empirical basis, he concluded that a necessary part of excellence was the notion of focused, repetitive practice. He described essential elements: a highly motivated individual can develop expertise through repetitive practice that also involves receiving feedback on performance, goal setting that continuously seeks to extend performance, individual coaching and practice occurring under different conditions. Like many approaches, this is not purely behaviourist in its approach, but there are key elements – 'well-defined learning objectives' and 'rigorous precise measurements' of demonstrated behaviours [4] – that align with behaviourism. See Box 2.1 for an example of how deliberate practice can be integrated into simulation educational design.

Box 2.1 Theory in Action: Patient-Focused Simulation

Deliberate practice, reflective practice and situated learning were developed in real rather than simulated settings and are appropriated with caution to the world of healthcare simulation. Drawing on these three theories, Roger Kneebone, a surgeon educator, and Debra Nestel, a communications educator, developed the concept of patient-focused simulation for learning procedural skills [11]. Patient-focused simulation involves a learner performing a procedural skill while working with a simulated (standardized) patient (SP) aligned with a task trainer (bench-top simulator). Kneebone and Nestel had noticed that teaching basic procedural skills on a task trainer was effective inasmuch as correct sequencing of psychomotor skills could be observed, but the experience was out of context. When the learner was required to perform the procedure on a patient in a clinical setting, the bench-top simulator experience alone was insufficient because it was not situated. That is, there was little resemblance to the setting in which the learner would be required to practise. Notably, there was no patient, no human interaction. Nestel and Kneebone argued that safe training approaches need to include ways in which learners can integrate complex sets of skills (psychomotor and professional) as they will be required in clinical settings. At a minimum, patient-focused simulation comprised a SP trained to respond as if undergoing the procedure in a simulated clinical setting. The learner in patient-focused simulation was offered the opportunity to perform the whole procedure in simulation and to receive feedback on their performance – from the SP and experienced clinicians and further individual reflection, to make sense of the experience from the learner's perspective. Elements of deliberate practice included motivating individuals, encouraging goal setting, multiple repetitions in different contexts and feedback. From situated learning, patient-focused simulation located the procedural skill in a clinical context with a SP; and from reflective practice, reflection-on-action was adopted, most commonly as facilitated dialogue between the learner, SP and observers after the simulation.

Constructivism and associated social learning theories

Constructivist theories of learning argue that individuals construct knowledge and meaning based on their experiences and ideas. Fosnot [6] claims that educators adopting constructivist theories enable learners to use 'concrete, contextually meaningful experience through which they can search for patterns, raise their own questions, and construct their own models, concepts, and strategies' (p. ix). Adopting this stance, educators may be seen to be orienting their role to that of facilitator rather than teacher. Using Sfard's metaphors [7], constructivists sit more comfortably within the metaphor of learning as participation than within that of learning as acquisition. Education is seen as what the learner can learn rather than what the teacher can teach.

Constructivism is an umbrella term for many theories that acknowledge the role of the learner in constructing their own meaning from experiences. *Cognitive* constructivism respects traditions of cognitivist theories, of acknowledging individuals' characteristics such as their stage of development, motivation, engagement and preferences for learning. *Social* constructivism emphasizes how understanding and meaning emerge from social encounters. Imagine a simulation educator who has been asked to design an activity for medical students to safely *put in a drip* (that is, establish a peripheral intravenous infusion, IVI). Adopting a constructivist stance, the educator is likely to use some of the following techniques:

- Finding out what other similar procedures students have been learning and how.
- Asking students about their relevant knowledge, prior experiences and practices relevant to IVI.
- Demonstrating, talking through and inviting questions from students on IVI performed on a task trainer.
- Encouraging students to set goals related to performing the IVI.
- Providing opportunities for students to perform the IVI on a task trainer.
- Providing opportunities for students to observe others performing the IVI on a task trainer and then share their observations.
- Providing opportunities for students to receive feedback on their performance on the task trainer from experts and peers.

CHAPTER 3

Historical practices in healthcare simulation: What we still have to learn

Harry Owen

KEY MESSAGES

- Immersive simulation was used in teaching obstetrics in many parts of Europe more than 250 years ago.

- Important concepts of simulation, including avoiding the learning curve on patients, repeated practice, expert supervision and feedback, preparing for rare events and simulator fidelity, were developed in the eighteenth century.

- Cadavers were widely used as obstetric and surgical simulators in the nineteenth century.

- A report of a US government audit of trauma care published in 1876 recommended the adoption of simulation in surgical training.

Overview

Simulation has been used in healthcare education for at least 1500 years and in the eighteenth, nineteenth and early twentieth centuries was widely used to help students learn new skills before performing procedures on patients. Often the use of simulation was a deliberate choice to reduce the risk of harm to patients, but in some areas, for example obstetrics training in the USA, simulation was used because there was very limited access to patients. Some of the early simulators were equivalent to task trainers and were used for learning basic principles and technical skills, but many simulators were developed for immersive training, where trainees could practise the management of rare conditions and serious complications. Simulation fidelity, the need to suspend disbelief and feedback were all well understood by the pioneers of simulation. Use of simulation in healthcare training declined significantly in the twentieth century and has only recently been rediscovered.

Introduction

The history of medicine has been a victim of the crowded medical curriculum and is no longer routinely taught. However, had we learnt from the pioneers of simulation in healthcare education, we would not have had to reinvent and rediscover how and when to use this most valuable training tool.

Background

Simulation has been used in training healthcare professionals for at least 1500 years, but the early examples of simulation were isolated geographically and temporally and were not sustained. This changed in the middle of the eighteenth century, when simulation became widely used in healthcare training in Europe and was then introduced to the USA. This was a time of great change in the world that would later be called the Age of Reason. Before this time the clergy preached the power of God and astrologers claimed that the stars could predict future events. However, when new ways of thinking were applied to daily living, it became apparent that most phenomena were governed by natural laws and that these could be deduced through experiment and careful observation. The natural philosophers in the universities of Europe described bodily systems as

Healthcare Simulation Education: Evidence, Theory and Practice, First Edition.
Edited by Debra Nestel, Michelle Kelly, Brian Jolly and Marcus Watson.
© 2018 John Wiley & Sons Ltd. Published 2018 by John Wiley & Sons Ltd.

machines governed by the same laws and considered that there was a scientific basis for diseases and their treatments. The beginning of modern medicine can be traced to the recognition that medication or a procedure can change the outcome of an abnormal condition. One of the first areas of healthcare to be affected by this was childbirth.

Simulation in obstetrics

In the seventeenth century, some physicians and surgeons applied themselves to what was originally called man-midwifery, before it became known as obstetrics. For example, William Harvey, better known for discovering the circulation, and who in 1649 also described how to make and use a pulse simulator and a percussion simulator for teaching, was a man-midwife. A man-midwife was often able to determine the cause of a prolonged labour and intervene as required, for which they received a higher fee than that of a midwife. Obstetric forceps were added to the armamentarium of man-midwives early in the eighteenth century. There was increased interest in midwifery as a profession and courses on obstetrics began to appear. In Paris, Grégoire the Younger was one of the first obstetrics teachers to use simulation to teach how to use forceps. Despite the slowness of travel at that time, Grégoire's course and his method of teaching were widely known and attracted many students.

In 1739 William Smellie, who had been practising as a surgeon-apothecary near Glasgow in Scotland, travelled to Paris on the advice of a friend to learn from Grégoire the Younger. Smellie had performed embryotomies to save mothers' lives when the pelvis was too small for the foetus to pass through, and he hoped that with forceps he could deliver a live child in such cases. Smellie was not impressed by the teaching he received from Grégoire, nor by the construction of the simulator, which was made of basket-work and covered with black leather. It contained a female pelvis and was used with a cadaver foetus, but, as Glaister notes [1], was too crude for Grégoire to use it to explain the difficulties that might be encountered (p. 26).

In Leiden, Herman Boerhaave had developed the concept of the hospital teaching round, which transformed medical education. Denman [2] records that in 1738, Sir Richard Manningham established the first obstetric teaching hospital in London (p. 567). Most women at that time gave birth at home and few were admitted to a lying-in hospital, but Manningham had a solution – simulation. In an advertisement for his course in the *London Evening Post* [3], Manningham explained how lectures on the theory and practice of midwifery would be enhanced by demonstrations and practice on simulators, so that 'each Pupil [will] become in a great measure proficient in his business before he attempts a real delivery' and 'all the inconveniences which might otherwise happen to women from pupils practising too early on real objects will be entirely prevented'.

Manningham actually developed two simulators for teaching, which he referred to as the 'glass machine' and the 'great machine'. The glass machine was used for

> illustration of the best and proficient methods of performing difficult deliveries with all possible ease and safety, a small glass matrix is contriv'd (in which is enclosed an artificial child) to be fix'd on ivory frames, imitating the various shapes of the bones forming the pelvis, in that every position the matrix or child can any way take and the hindrance either may meet from the said bones and the easiest and most effectual ways of performing all difficult deliveries, (as is taught on the great machine) together with the realms of the rules, will hereby in a most instructive manner be beautifully and clearly represented to the eye.

The 'great machine' was a life-size simulator 'made on the bones or skeleton of a woman, with an artificial matrix [uterus]' that was used for 'the performance of deliveries of all kinds, with the utmost decency and dexterity'. Manningham observed that to become proficient students needed repeated practice under supervision on this machine, 'where every case that can happen may be represented, and repeated as often as we see necessary'. He explained [4] that the cognitive load was managed by teaching 'first the most natural and easy; and then those which are more difficult; and lastly, to the most difficult and praeternatural Deliveries that can possibly happen' (p. 5). He was not the first to demonstrate birth on a simulator, as Van Hoorn had used a simulator with an artificial foetus to demonstrate childbirth during lectures at the beginning of the eighteenth century, but Manningham was the first to integrate simulation into a clinical teaching programme, and he deserves to be recognized for this.

It was Grégoire's simulator that gave Smellie the idea that simulators 'should so exactly imitate real women and children as to exhibit to the learner all the difficulties that happen in midwifery'. Smellie established an obstetric practice in London and taught both man-midwives and female midwives. None of Smellie's simulators has survived, but there are several descriptions of them, which attest that they were lifelike in form, feel and function. Camper wrote they were 'made out of leather with such remarkable skill that not only is the structure as natural as possible but the necessary functions of parturition are performed by working models' [5].

Smellie recognized that few labours required active intervention, so students would encounter few if any of the many complications they might meet later in clinical practice and be expected to manage. He suggested [6]:

> In order to acquire a more perfect idea of the art, he ought to perform with his own hands upon proper machines, contrived to convey a just notion of all the difficulties to be met with in every kind of labour; by which means he will learn how to use the forceps and crotchets with more dexterity, be accustomed to the turning of children, and consequently be more capable of acquitting himself in troublesome cases that may happen to him when he comes to practise among women; he should also embrace every occasion of being present at real labours. (p. 429)

In the middle of the eighteenth century simulation was also used in Germany [7] and Italy [8] and soon afterwards was introduced into the USA [9].

However, the expansion in midwifery training took place in the cities of Europe and left rural areas underserved. In the second half of the eighteenth century a national rural simulation-based midwifery training programme was developed in France by Angélique Marguerite Le Boursier du Coudray. There were actually two courses delivered in regional centres across France: one to train new midwives and another train-the-trainer course for rural surgeons. Students attended lectures in the mornings and practised on simulators in the afternoons. Writing about her midwifery teaching [10], du Coudray noted: 'We have the advantage of students practicing on the machine and performing all the deliveries imaginable. Therein lies the principle merit of this invention' (p. 16). Simulators were left at each centre for the surgeons to teach new midwives and for annual refresher courses. Simulators

made of better materials or with a system of sponges that could dispense clear or opaque red liquids could be ordered at extra expense. Students were taught the importance of calling for help in emergencies and of the handover procedures (p. 70). This programme was very successful and was copied, which led to an industry in manufacturing and repairing obstetric simulators.

Use of simulation in obstetrics and midwifery expanded in the nineteenth century and simulator design reflected new techniques and procedures. A change in position of the body for delivery, from upright to supine, is evident in the design of obstetric simulators. When Pinard established guidelines to determine orientation of the foetus by external palpation [11], a simulator with a rubber abdominal wall was developed to practise the skill.

A low point in medical education was the use of female cadavers as obstetric simulators, which began in Vienna and spread across Europe and to the USA. Unfortunately, the transmission of infection was poorly understood and this practice resulted in tens of thousands of deaths. Only now is simulation used to promote and improve hand hygiene. Another low point was the use of the poor as teaching material. Osiander in Göttingen called them 'living phantoms' [12] and he used forceps for teaching more often than was clinically necessary to assist delivery.

Many medical schools in the USA adopted obstetric simulation at this time (Figure 3.1), although sometimes this was to remedy a shortage of patients. This was the case at Long Island College Hospital (LICH), Brooklyn, New York [13], but simulation was used extensively 'so that notwithstanding the paucity of clinical material, when a Long Island man was confronted with an obstetric proposition, he was qualified to deal with it' (p. 5). A building at LICH that opened in 1897 included four simulation rooms with facilities for observation. Also, a dynamometer was used with the simulators to measure the force being applied to them. In an article on the teaching in this simulation suite it was noted that '[t]he student is drilled in diagnostic methods and in the various obstetric manoeuvres' [14].

At the Obstetric Institute of Philadelphia, medical students were paired up with pupil nurses for simulation training. These teams were then expected to demonstrate in front of the whole class every manipulation and operation necessary from the beginning of labour, including washing and dressing the baby and putting

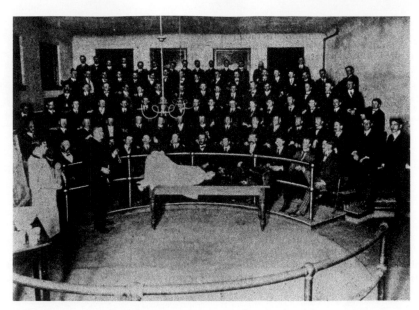

Figure 3.1 Mannequin-based obstetric teaching at the Chattanooga Medical College, circa 1903. Source: Courtesy US National Library of Medicine.

it to the mother's breast. Students had to demonstrate proficiency on a patient simulator before they were given permission to perform those procedures on patients.

Several studies published early in the twentieth century identified a need for obstetric simulation in US medical curricula. For example, a report by the Committee on Maternal Welfare of the American Association of Obstetricians, Gynecologists and Abdominal Surgeons observed that didactic instruction was not sufficient and that practical skills needed to be taught to small classes first on a simulator and later by the combined use of simulator and patient. One of the most influential reports of the time, by Abraham Flexner [15], was quite silent on the topic. Simulation in obstetric training underwent a significant decline in the second half of the twentieth century.

Simulation in bronchoscopy

Anaesthesia was discovered in the middle of the nineteenth century and this facilitated the development of many new surgical procedures. Up to the end of the century inhalation of a foreign body had serious consequences, but that was completely changed by Gustav Killian's invention of bronchoscopy. Killian developed the technique on cadavers and in 1897 used it to examine the bronchial tree of a live subject and to remove foreign bodies. Two years later he demonstrated the technique on what were called 'living simulators' at a conference in Germany. There was intense interest in bronchoscopy, but operating the long, slender instruments was hard to learn. In a lecture given in 1902, Killian observed: 'Their manipulation at so great a depth is not an easy matter, but may be learned and practised on a phantom. I have constructed one for this purpose' [16].

Early in the twentieth century simulation was widely recommended for learning bronchoscopy. Jackson, for example, recommended a few hundred hours' practice on a simulator to develop the required skills [17], and Walgett advised [18]: 'When the nature of the foreign body is known, actual practice should be made with its duplicate placed in the phantom' (p. 313).

Jackson included a chapter on acquiring skills in a book on per-oral endoscopy published in 1922 [17], in which he recommended practice using the equipment on a 'Rubber-tube Manikin', cadavers and dogs. The rubber-tube mannequin was readily available and

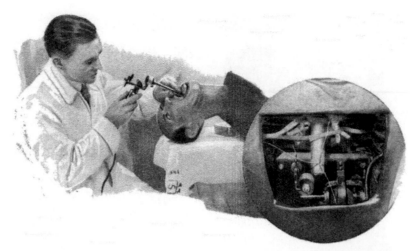

Figure 3.2 A per-oral endoscopy simulator developed in the Hajek Clinic in Vienna [20]. The text explained: 'This robot makes a nervous patient for the medical student and lights up or rings a bell if the probe goes right or wrong. At right, the insides of the model that cause it to respond to stimuli.'

was very useful for learning to use the equipment. When endoscopy was performed on a cadaver, Jackson recommended that the whole surgical team, including the assistant who holds the head and the one who passes the instruments, should practise together, as 'in no other way can the pupil be taught to avoid killing his patient'. He added that '[l]aryngeal growths may be simulated, foreign body problems created and their mechanical difficulties solved and practice work with the forceps and tube perfected' (ch. 11). Jackson noted that it was necessary to maintain flexibility of the cadaver and recommended a special embalming solution containing arsenic and alcohol. Bronchoscopy on dogs provided experience of the procedure on a live subject with respiration, cardiac pulsation and secretions, but Jackson reported the need to suspend disbelief, or 'the endoscopist will lose much of the value of his dog practice if he fails to regard the dog as a child'.

In 1928, Alper described 'a breathing, pulsating man-sized phantom for bronchoscopic and esophagoscopic manipulations' that had been developed in the Hajek clinic in Vienna (Figure 3.2). This simulator provided feedback to the endoscopist and it was later reported [19] that the simulator was useful in medical education because:

- It could be operated on at convenient times for any number of diseases.
- A novice can operate on the simulator for serious conditions without increased risk to patients.

- The same operation can be repeated many times on the same day.
- It can be used to practise treating patients with an infectious disease without spreading the illness.
- Unusual cases and their treatment can be demonstrated and practised.

Unfortunately, it seems that the use of simulation in learning bronchoscopy declined in the second half of the twentieth century. A review of complications from bronchoscopy in a US teaching hospital published in 1978 revealed a higher rate of complications than was generally reported [21], and this was attributed to procedures performed by trainees who were inexperienced. A study of bronchoscopy training published in 2006 [22] confirmed an increased rate of complications among novice bronchoscopists. At the institution concerned, trainees received lectures on bronchoscopy but no formal training on a simulator, even though one was available. It was concluded that '[f]uture research is needed to determine the role of advanced educational techniques, including the use of simulators, in facilitating bronchoscopy education' [22].

The lost history of simulation in healthcare

Over 250 years ago it was acknowledged that risk of harm to patients could be greatly reduced by having students and trainees learn procedures through simulation. It was also recognized that simulation could be used to prepare for uncommon conditions that are difficult to manage and to learn new procedures. In 1876, the US government published a national audit of treatment of abdominal injuries during the American Civil War. One of the recommendations made in the report [23] was that newer and 'more complicated methods and modifications … should not be attempted on the living subject until the operator has acquired some experience by practicing, as M. Fano used to require his pupils to do, either using the fingers of a glove, or, better still, upon a recent subject, or on intestines placed in a manikin' (p. 121). The introduction of laparoscopic surgery in the last quarter of the twentieth century was associated with increased injuries to patients and has been described as 'the biggest unaudited free for all in the history of surgery' [24].

Around 100 years ago it was recommended that healthcare teams should practise together using simulation. Quite recently training courses using simulation have been re-established in many healthcare disciplines, but simulation has not been formally integrated into training and most procedures are still learnt on patients. It was in the middle of the nineteenth century that Semmelweis discovered that using cadavers as obstetric simulators was the source of puerperal fever then endemic in the main hospital in Vienna [25]. Many of his colleagues refused to integrate his methods to control the infection in their practice, and Semmelweis responded by calculating the number of deaths they caused through their indifference to improving patient care. Today we could calculate the harm and costs arising from training on patients instead of on simulators, since it appears that we have not learnt much from the historical practices of healthcare simulation. The work of the pioneers of simulation should not be ignored and we should use their legacy to the fullest possible extent.

References

1 Glaister, J. Dr., (1894) *William Smellie and his contemporaries; a contribution to the history of midwifery in the eighteenth century,* Glasgow, Maclehose.

2 Denman T. *An introduction to the practice of midwifery.* New York: G. & C. & H. Carvill [u.a.]; 1782.

3 Manningham R. Lectures advertisement. London Evening Post. 1740; p. 4.

4 Manningham, R. (1744) *An abstract of midwifry,* T. Gardner, London.

5 Van Heiningen, T. (2014) *Wouter Van Doeveren and Petrus Camper in Paris: travel diaries kept in the years 1752–1753, 1777 & 1787 and related correspondence,* Den Haag, Digitaal Wetenchapshistorisch Centrum.

6 Smellie, W. (1766) *A treatise on the theory and practice of ,idwifery,* 5th edn, London.

7 Börner, F. (1752) *Die gebährende Frau,* Frankfurt.

8 Fabbri GB. Antico museo ostetrico di Giovanni Antonio Galli, restauro fatto alle sue operazioni in plastica e nuova conferma della suprema importanza dell'ostetricia sperimentale: discorso letto nella sessione del 2 maggio 1872 dell'Accademia delle Scienze dell'Istituto di Bologna. Bologna: Tipi Gamberini E Parmeggiani; **1872**. pp. 129–166.

9 Owen, H. (2016) *Simulation in healthcare education: an extensive history,* Springer, New York.

10 Gelbert, N.R. (1998) *The king's midwife: a history and mystery of Madame du Coudray,* University of California Press, Berkeley, CA.

11 Dunn, P. (2006) Adolphe Pinard (1844–1934) of Paris and intrauterine paediatric care. *Arch Dis Child Fetal Neonatal Ed.,* **91**, F231–F232. doi: 10.1136/adc.2005.074518

12 Schlumbohm, J. (2012) *Lebendige Phantome – ein Entbindungshospital und seine Patientinnen 1751–1830,* Goettingen, Wallstein.

13 Polak, J.O. (1925) The history and development of the Department of Obstetrics and Gynecology. *Long Island Coll Alumni J.,* **2**, 4–6.

14 Jewett, C. (1905) Teaching methods in gynecology and obstetrics. *Brooklyn Med J,* **19** (9), 337–9.

15 Flexner, A. (1910) *Medical education in the United States and Canada: a report to the Carnegie Foundation for the Advancement of Teaching.*

16 Killian, G. (1902) On direct endoscopy of the upper air passages and oesophagus; its diagnostics and the therapeutic value in the search for and removal of foreign bodies. *BMJ,* **2** (2174), 569–571.

17 Jackson, C. (1922) *Bronchoscopy and esophagoscopy: a manual of peroral endoscopy and laryngeal surgery.*

18 Waggett E. *Direct laryngoscopy, tracheoscopy, bronchoscopy, oesphagoscopy and gastroscopy.* In: Allbutt C, Rolleston H, editors. *A system of medicine by many writers.* 1910. pp. 299–322.

19 Unknown. Vienna Robot so human it suffers from illness. Milwaukee Sentinel; 1930:19.

20 Unknown. Young doctors' robot rings bell at error. Pop Sci. 1930:**30**.

21 Dreisin, R., Albert, R., Talley, P. *et al.* (1978) Flexible fiberoptic bronchoscopy in the teaching hospital: yield and complications. *Chest,* **74** (2), 144–9.

making and prioritizing within the team – creating maximum learning possibilities.

Strategies for managing realism and meaningfulness to promote learning

We propose strategies for simulation educators before, during and after simulations to manage realism and meaningfulness to promote learning (Figure 4.2). *Before* the simulation, when inviting participants it can be made clear that learning will be in a simulated environment. Immediately before the simulation, educators can identify features and functions of a simulator that are similar and those that are different to reality and how this will be managed. Participants can be asked about their feelings towards the simulation and what they are hoping to achieve. Simulation educators can draw on real clinical events in designing scenarios that are aligned with participants' needs. *During* the simulation, educators can maintain the fiction contract and conduct scenarios in a realistic way. They can encourage discussion of safe and unsafe practices during debriefings. *After* the simulation, participants can be asked about realism and meaningfulness during the evaluation to inform faculty development and scenario design.

Examples of realism in healthcare simulation

Here we share four examples of different simulation modalities and associated considerations of realism from the perspective of simulation educators.

Example 4.1: simulated patients – realism in role portrayal

SPs are people well trained to portray patients. Many variables influence their level of realism during simulations. This includes casting – needs to be credible; the scenario – needs to be believable; the learner's task – needs to be appropriate for the SP role; and the SP portrayal – needs to be accurate, have internal consistency and be emotionally flexible. In an effort to achieve *standardization* for exams, SP realism can be compromised, as the desire to provide every candidate with the same experience takes precedence over authentic portrayal. However, designing SP roles that are based on real patients and offering rigorous training for portrayal can address some of these issues. Nestel et al. [23] describe a study in which they used a template to interview patients who had recently undergone procedural skills in the emergency department. Based on the interviews, SP roles were developed that mirrored the real patients' experiences and included their phrases and emotions. In another unpublished study funded by

Before			During			After
Inviting learners	Developing faculty	Designing scenarios	Creating an engaging learning environment	Implementing scenarios	Maintaining an engaging learning environment	Evaluating simulations
Brief orientation to simulation	Selection and development	Based on detailed task analysis	Establishing fiction contract at course beginning	Task-appropriate conduct	Maintaining fiction contract during debriefings	Ask for learners' feedback on realism
Email highlighting the idea of simulation training	*Training simulated patients in role portrayal*	*Selective abstraction during distributed simulation*	*Highlighting collaborative learning*	*Using 'real' time*	*Acknowledging learners' perceptions*	*Web-based questionnaire*

Figure 4.2 Considerations for realism in healthcare simulations. The text in italics offers examples of actions to address elements of realism before, during and after simulations.

Imperial College London as a Teaching Development Grant and led by Debra Nestel, patients from a general practice setting who had complex histories were interviewed and their stories and experiences documented as a *narrative*, which was then used as the basis for SP roles. In this study, SPs met with the real patients whose stories they were portraying. This was salutary for the SPs, as they connected directly with those whom they were *re-presenting*, a powerful reminder of the meaning of their work.

Example 4.2: real rather than compressed time – learning cardiopulmonary resuscitation

Krogh et al. [24] described how when attending *code blue* (cardiac arrest) emergency calls it was noticed that junior doctors were not keeping the recommended two minutes of cardiopulmonary resuscitation (CPR) between rhythm control/defibrillation. A study was undertaken of advanced life support (ALS) training to investigate whether shortened CPR cycles could be the source of lack of adherence to the ALS guidelines. Participants took part in a one-day ALS course where they were randomized to attend simulation scenarios using real-time CPR (120 seconds [s]) or shortened-time CPR cycles (30–45 s). Adherence to time was measured 1 and 12 weeks after the course using the European Resuscitation Council's Cardiac Arrest Simulation Test. The results showed that the real-time CPR group adhered significantly better to the recommended 120 s CPR cycles [24]. In this study, real rather than compressed time was a relevant and important part of overall realism (Figure 4.2). The risk of *negative learning* needs to be considered in the design of learning activities.

Example 4.3: distributed simulation – mobile immersive clinical environments

In this example we consider the setting of the simulation in which *good enough* realism is acceptable. Kneebone et al. [25] describe *Distributed Simulation* (DS), an immersive inflatable enclosure. The DS is the product of a team of industrial designers, prosthetic makers, special effects artists, information technologists, educationalists, simulated patients and clinicians. An active design process was used to identify the salient environmental features for re-creating in a simulated setting. Participants in the simulation use their own mental models to translate images of clinical environments to the simulated one. By including only minimal cues rather than everything in the environment, the functional flexibility of the DS can be increased. By the inclusion of different props and different photographic backdrops, it can be used for emergency department, intensive care, recovery room, operating theatre and more. The DS can be used in any room of sufficient size to take the enclosure. It inflates in a few minutes and equipment from the local site can be readily included in the DS. In some ways, the DS sits between the static simulation centre and simulations in clinical settings. It is currently used for teaching, learning and research activities.

Example 4.4: cross-training – rotating positions to enhance perspective taking

The final example describes a specific team training intervention, cross-training, in which realism is temporarily reduced for the sake of allowing team members to perceive and understand each other's perspectives and thus enhancing their overall understanding of the team's task. During cross-training, team members rotate roles [26, 27]. For example, a nurse takes on the role of an attending physician and an attending physician takes on the role of a nurse. The advantage of this training intervention is that it significantly facilitates the development of team interaction mental models; that is, the shared understanding among team members of how to work together [28]. A risk of cross-training is that participants may feel overwhelmed and experience too much stress, for example due to lack of knowledge or experience with the unfamiliar role. *Lighter* versions of cross-training, such as watching training videotapes modelling each others' positions rather than fully engaging in one another's roles, seem equally effective [28]. Alternatively, inviting a participant in an anaesthesia crisis resource management course (perhaps an anaesthetic trainee) to participate in the scenario as an additional, *embedded* simulated surgeon, being briefed just to observe the case from the surgeon's perspective, seems beneficial as well.

provide a more robust assessment of the strengths and weaknesses of new technologies and are likely to predict barriers to the introduction of new technologies and practices.

In well-designed simulations, the experience can be controlled and rare clinical events can be reliably integrated. As with training, the use of debriefing allows for a deeper understanding of individual and team experiences. Debriefing cannot be as easily conducted for clinical trials of new technologies and/or procedures due to ongoing patient and operational needs. In clinical trials of new technologies and/or procedures, patient safety concerns may prohibit novices from participating. The use of simulation does however allow for clinicians of all levels of expertise to participate. This is very important in understanding the different training requirements for novices to learn and experienced clinicians to adapt to new practices. Such simulation can also be used to identify cultural barriers to the adoption of new technologies and processes, which may differ across both professional groups and levels of skill.

As simulation can play a role in patient flow redesign [10], simulation can also play a role in the design of new technologies. For example, to ensure that patients who deteriorate receive appropriate and timely care, the right tools, systems of escalation and training are required. Historically healthcare failed to recognize that patient charts are actually clinical decision support tools that should be empirically evaluated for their effectiveness. In 2009 the Australian Commission on Safety and Quality in Healthcare commissioned work on the design and evaluation of charts to support recognition and response to deterioration. The use of simulation was combined with human factors methodologies to analyse, design and evaluate the effectiveness of charts for individual and team requirements (micro and meso). Empirical studies have since demonstrated that these processes have developed a more effective adult deterioration detection system than the charts already in clinical use [14]. A further study has shown that the design process trumped health professionals' prior chart experience and demonstrates that investment in the design of clinical support tools is more effective than good training [15]. In modified versions of the charts, clinical evaluation indicated a reduction in cardiac arrest events [16]. Investment in simulation to support the design and evaluation of healthcare tools and processes

is likely to provide greater returns than simulation focused on training.

The process used in the micro simulations for the design of the adult deterioration detection system has evolved into simulation rapid prototyping (SRP). SRP is an extension of existing human factors design methodologies and healthcare debriefing techniques, and has now been used to address individual, team and organizational needs for a range of technologies. In a 2014 example, SRP was used in the bedside observation monitoring and escalation proof of concept that examined the potential of two existing electronic deterioration detection systems to be used in a major hospital and health services. The purpose of simulations was to identify quality improvement opportunities and staff acceptance of using the new technologies, rather than comparing the two systems.

The process simulated a close observation unit to examine what would need to change at the micro, meso and macro levels of the hospital and health services in order to move to electronic patient monitoring. The simulations were undertaken by small teams of nurses from the different hospitals across the service, while the debriefing included the simulated patient and observers from all aspects of the hospital service, including medicine and allied health executives and information systems teams. The debriefing addressed the difference in experience between the paper-based and electronic systems and also drew on the broader observer group. This enabled sharing of how this would affect their work and the hospital and health service's existing systems to support the uptake of electronic systems. Unique to this study were the systems developers, who were able to watch their systems in action in the simulations and debriefing via a remote video feed. This arrangement allowed wider participation in the final discussion about the flexibility of their systems to address micro, meso and macro issues identified in the scenarios and debriefing.

As the simulations were designed to analyse existing practices and predict the strengths and weaknesses of moving to electronic practices, the focus was on discovery, not control. The systems developers were able to provide a variety of hardware and evolving software during the three days over which their system was used. This allowed both participants in the simulation and observer groups to better envisage existing barriers and solutions required if the service were to move to electronic bedside observation monitoring and escalation systems. Issues identified included hardware selection, user interfaces, training requirements, processes of care and information technology (IT) infrastructure. Although many issues were identified at all levels (micro, meso and macro) of the healthcare service, participants' acceptance of the potential for electronic systems dramatically shifted as a result of the simulations. Such uses of simulations are not experiments, but rather opportunities to explore the potential for different ways of delivering care. Unlike an expert working group, SRP provides rich experiences, which allow a greater exploration of the possible solutions rather than relying on opinions based on clinicians' experiences.

If proof-of-concept simulations where the focus is on understanding the needs of patients, clinicians and the healthcare system and not on the procurement of a system are undertaken, the potential of new technologies and practices can be engaged at appropriate times and with a better understanding of what is likely to change throughout the system. The involvement of systems developers in SRP allowed them to better understand healthcare systems requirements and potential barriers that needed to be addressed in order for their systems to work effectively in patient care. Simulation has the potential to provide better developmental environments than even the eventual clinical setting, because of the ability to generate situations reliably and to explore where the boundaries of safe practice lie for existing and new practices.

SRP still has limits; such processes require significant work in the development of the scenarios. For example, the bedside observation monitoring and escalation systems took five weeks to develop and deliver with a large team. The skills required to undertake such proofs of concept are expertise in simulation, human factors, systems design and significant experience of the healthcare system. To capitalize on such investments, processes such as SRP would be more effective if they were used to inform computer models in order to aggregate knowledge capture and visualize potential future systems.

Conclusion

Healthcare simulation will play an expanding role in training and must go beyond the focus of developing competent clinicians to developing proficient teams who work in resilient systems. To do this we need to use simulation to understand human system integration at the cognitive and social levels of interaction in healthcare. Using a framework to scaffold different simulations may help to bridge the divide between training and design at all levels of healthcare. The use of discrete event simulation to improve macro processes of care should be achievable by most simulation providers. Nevertheless, as technology continues to grow exponentially, the healthcare simulation community needs to develop the capacity to conduct predictive simulation to understand how to adapt to new technologies and, even more importantly, to help design the right technologies, processes and training to ensure safe, high-quality care.

References

1 Vincent, C., Aylin, P., Franklin, B.D. *et al.* (2008) Is health care getting safer? *BMJ*, **337** (7680), 1205–7.

2 Wachter, R.M. (2010) Patient safety at ten: unmistakable progress, troubling gaps. *Health Aff*, **29** (1), 165–73.

3 Kohn, L.T., Corrigan, J.M. and Donaldson, M.S. (eds) (1999) *To err is human: building a safer health system*, National Academy Press, Washington, DC.

4 Swan N, Balendra J. Wasted. Four Corners. 28 Sept 2015. Available at: http://www.abc.net.au/4corners/stories/2015/09/28/4318883.htm

5 Carayon, P. and Wood, K.E. (2010) Patient safety: the role of human factors and systems engineering. *Stud Health Technol Inform.*, **153**, 23–46.

6 Khosravi, A., Nahavandi, S. and Creighton, D. (2009) Interpreting and modeling baggage handling system as a system of systems. *IEEE International Conference on Industrial Technology*, 1–6.

7 Arora, S. and Sevdalis, N. (2008) HOSPEX and concepts of simulation. *JR Army Medical Corps*, **154** (3), 202–5.

8 Sutton, R.M., Niles, D., Meaney, P.A. *et al.* (2011) Low-dose, high-frequency CPR training improves skill retention of in-hospital pediatric providers. *Pediatrics*, **128** (1), e145–e151. doi: 10.1542/peds.2010-2105

9 Andreatta, P., Saxton, E., Thompson, M. *et al.* (2011) Simulation-based mock codes significantly correlate with improved pediatric patient cardiopulmonary arrest survival rates. *Pediatr Crit Care Med*, **12** (1), 33–8.

10 Brazil V, Baldwin M, Dooris M, Muller H, Cullen L. 'Stemi-sim' – a 'process of care' simulation can help improve door to balloon times for patients with ST elevation myocardial infarction. *SimHealth Sydney*. 2012;10–13 Sept.

CHAPTER 6

Strategies for research in healthcare simulation

Debra Nestel & Michelle Kelly

KEY MESSAGES

- Healthcare simulation research is diverse and draws on many disciplines.
- Research strategies are important in developing programmes of research.
- Professional associations and other communities of practice often support strategic approaches to healthcare simulation research.
- Research strategies may offer researchers guidance in identifying topics and approaches for investigation.
- Multidisciplinary research is likely to offer insights to the many questions posed by healthcare simulation researchers.

Overview

This chapter commences with a status report on health professions educational research generally and then quickly focuses on simulation. Although educational research features here, this does not diminish the importance of other types of healthcare simulation research. The chapter then explores the activities of professional societies and special interest groups in setting research agendas, hosting research summits, establishing research networks and supporting peer-reviewed journals focused on the dissemination of healthcare simulation practice and outcomes. Brief reference is made to the need for properly funded healthcare simulation research.

Introduction

The vibrancy of the healthcare simulation research community is manifested in many ways. This chapter explores the activities of professional societies and other communities of practice (e.g. special interest groups) in setting research agendas, hosting research summits and facilitating professional development in research skills. Additional activities include supporting peer-reviewed journals focused on healthcare simulation, enabling the dissemination of research, innovation and scholarship, all intended to advance healthcare simulation. We place a strong emphasis on research related to the role of simulation in the context of health professions education. However, we acknowledge that healthcare simulation research has a much broader reach and role.

Reviews of health professions educational research usually conclude with the need for improved rigour in research, and with the claim that studies often have no theoretical framework, weak research design and fail to measure meaningful impact. A commonly used framework for the evaluation of educational interventions is Kirkpatrick's model [1], which has been modified for interprofessional education [2]. However, this model has also been critiqued in part for its simplistic approach to measuring change [3]. Furthermore, the health professions educational community's heavy reliance on a single approach disregards the rich discipline of programme evaluation [4, 5]. The distinction between *evaluation* and *research* is also important and detailed discussion is beyond the scope of this chapter; suffice it to

Healthcare Simulation Education: Evidence, Theory and Practice, First Edition.
Edited by Debra Nestel, Michelle Kelly, Brian Jolly and Marcus Watson.
© 2018 John Wiley & Sons Ltd. Published 2018 by John Wiley & Sons Ltd.

acknowledge that simple evaluation-orientated studies are usually not considered research. Health professions educational research has often been judged according to an 'ideal' model of research in the physical sciences [6]. However, there is increasing acceptance of research models from the social sciences as offering valuable approaches to exploring the complexity of learning and practice [6–8]. Focusing on simulation-based education, a critical review of published research targeting the years 2003–09 identified 'twelve features and best practices' [9]. For each feature and practice, the authors also identified gaps in understanding and posed questions for researchers to answer. As an orientation to the field, the paper is well worth reading.

As an indirect approach to improving the rigour of healthcare simulation research, Cheng et al. have published reporting guidelines [10]. They surveyed experts and established a consensus panel, both of whom considered extensions to the existing Consolidated Standards of Reporting Trials (CONSORT) and Strengthening the Reporting of Observational Studies in Epidemiology (STROBE) statements. This resulted in the article's publication, with a notable advancement in the detailed reporting of key elements for simulation research such as participant orientation, simulator type, simulator environment, simulation event/scenario, instructional design (for educational interventions) or exposure (for simulation as investigative methodology) and feedback and/or debriefing. These guidelines are intended to facilitate meaningful comparisons of study outcomes through more complete and consistent reporting.

McGaghie et al. mount strong arguments for translational research in healthcare simulation [11]. This is the *bench to bedside* notion associated with biomedical and clinical sciences. There are multiple levels, referred to as T1 (e.g. research that measures performance during the simulation scenario), T2 (e.g. performance in clinical settings) and T3 (e.g. economic evaluations and sustainability) [12]. Much healthcare simulation research is at T1 and T2 and there are some examples at T3. Given that the activities of the healthcare simulation research community are so diverse, we believe that it is also important to value theoretical research, since this will aid in understanding and insight, furthering innovation, advancing simulation practices and indirectly improving patient outcomes. Research is also likely to be multidisciplinary because of the complexity of the questions being asked in relation to healthcare practices.

Professional societies and research strategies

Establishing an overarching strategy can be useful in guiding the development of programmes of research. A strategic approach may build speciality expertise (content, methodology and methods), lead to opportunities to attract funding through clarity of vision, facilitate multisite research, guide new researchers and offer insight to potential collaborators from within and external to the healthcare simulation community. Examples of these strategic approaches are shared in this chapter and we direct readers to the full papers for more detail.

The earliest documented strategic approach that we found was from the Society for Academic Emergency Medicine (SAEM) Simulation Task Force, which was developed in 2006. The agenda proposed studies on reflective and experiential learning, behavioural and team training, procedural simulation, computer screen-based simulation, the use of simulation for evaluation and testing, and special topics in emergency medicine [13]. Although the process of development of the agenda is unclear, the paper presents insightful research questions, many of which have relevance a decade later.

The second example is from Issenberg et al. in 2011, who report on an Utstein-style meeting designed to establish a research agenda for simulation-based healthcare education [14]. Twenty researchers from different health professions and countries were invited to a two-day meeting in Copenhagen. Working through a specific process, they identified three main themes for research questions:
- Learning acquisition, retention of skills and cognitive load
- Debriefing
- Learner characteristics

Subthemes included instructional design, outcome measurement and translational research. Box 6.1 includes examples of questions associated with the first main theme on *learning acquisition, retention of skills* and *cognitive load*. The outcome of this meeting informed the content of the research summit outlined next, so an immediate and direct impact was realized.

Box 6.1 Examples of questions from the research agenda for simulation-based healthcare education [14]

Theme: Learning acquisition, retention of skills and cognitive load

- How do theories of learning and teaching inform the design of simulation interventions (e.g. frequency, timing and deliberate practice)?
- How do theories of cognitive load inform the design and structure of simulation programmes, courses and concrete scenarios based on the complexity of tasks required for learners to acquire and maintain?
- How do different simulation modalities and their contextualized use affect skill development and retention?

A research consensus summit of the Society for Simulation in Healthcare (SSH) comprises our third example [15]. The summit was intended to identify the current *state of the science* of simulation-related research, provide guidance on the use of simulation, broaden the scope of simulation research, offer breadth in research topics and methods and foreground the value of research to the wider international healthcare simulation community. Ten topics were identified for further investigation by small groups of diverse, international health professionals and other disciplinary researchers, for wider discussion at the summit. Topics included the role of simulation in procedural skills, team training and human factors. Other groups focused on research methods and assessment of learning outcomes, and on the assessment and regulation of healthcare professionals, instructional science, systems designs, translational patient outcomes and reporting of simulation research. Many of the topic reports proceeded to publication [16–18]. A second research summit is scheduled for 2017.

The fourth example is from a specialist professional community, Stefanidis et al.'s 2012 report on research priorities in surgical simulation for the twenty-first century [19]. A driver for their strategy was the apparent lack of coordination and focus of surgical simulation research. Using a Delphi method, members of the US-based Association for Surgical Education (ASE) submitted 226 research questions about simulation, which were subsequently reduced to 74 and then rated for priority. Categories of questions covered simulation effectiveness/outcomes, team training, performance assessment and credentialling, curriculum, simulator/simulation validity and resources/personnel (Box 6.2). The highest-ranked question was: *Does simulator training lead to improved patient outcomes, safety, and quality of care?* Three years later, members of the ASE Simulation Committee undertook literature reviews addressing each question and reported progress in the areas of skills assessment, curriculum development, debriefing and decision making in surgery [20]. Despite being the highest-ranked question in the first agenda, the impact of simulation training on patient outcomes remains a challenging issue to address and is reported as a major focus for future research. In 2015 Johnston et al. commended the efforts that researchers have made towards T2- and T3-level studies [20] and, like researchers before them [11, 12], acknowledged the challenges associated with research of this nature.

Box 6.2 Ten questions from the research agenda for surgical simulation by Stefanidis et al. and Johnston et al. [19, 20]

---

1 Does simulator training lead to improved patient outcomes, safety and quality of care?
2 Does training on simulators transfer to improved clinical performance?
3 Does documented simulator competence equal clinical competence?
4 What are the best methods/metrics to assess technical and non-technical performance on simulators and in the operating room?
5 What are the performance criteria that surgical trainees need to achieve to be competent based on their training level (on a national level)?
6 What is the role of simulation for certification of residents and practising surgeons?
7 How can we use simulation to teach and assess judgement and decision making in routine and crisis situations?
8 What type and method of feedback are most effective to improve performance on simulators?
9 How should a simulator curriculum be designed and evaluated?
10 How do we train and assess teams effectively using simulation?

The fifth example is from a national professional society. In 2013, Simulation Australasia hosted a research

social care, UK Centre for the Advancement of Interprofessional Education/British Educational Research Association, London.

3 Bates, R. (2004) A critical analysis of evaluation practice: the Kirkpatrick model and the principle of beneficence. *Eval Program Plann.*, **27**, 341–7.

4 Fitzpatrick, J., Sanders, J. and Worthen, B. (2011) *Program evaluation: alternative approaches and practical guidelines*, 4th edn, Pearson Education, Upper Saffle River, NJ.

5 Alkin, M. (ed.) (2013) *Evaluation roots: a wider perspective of theorists' views and influences*, 2nd edn, Sage, Berkeley, CA.

6 Regehr, G. (2010) It's NOT rocket science: rethinking our metaphors for research in health professions education. *Med Educ.*, **44**, 31–9.

7 Traynor, R. and Eva, K.W. (2010) The evolving field of medical education research. *Biochem Mol Biol Educ*, **36** (4), 211–15.

8 Hodges, B. and Kuper, A. (2012) Theory and practice in the design and conduct of graduate medical education. *Acad Med*, **87** (1), 25–33.

9 McGaghie, W.C., Issenberg, S.B., Petrusa, E.R. and Scalese, R.J. (2010) A critical review of simulation-based medical education research: 2003–2009. *Med Educ*, **44** (1), 50–63. doi: 10.1111/j.1365-2923.2009.03547.x

10 Cheng, A., Kessler, D., Mackinnon, R. *et al.* (2016) Reporting guidelines for health care simulation research: extensions to the CONSORT and STROBE statements. *Adv Simul.*, **1**. doi: 10.1186/s41077-016-0025-y

11 McGaghie, W.C., Draycott, T.J., Dunn, W.F. *et al.* (2011) Evaluating the impact of simulation on translational patient outcomes. *Simul Healthc.*, **6** (Suppl), S42–7. doi: 10.1097/SIH.0b013e318222fde9

12 Gaba, D. (2015) Expert's corner: research in healthcare simulation, in *Defining excellence in simulation programs* (eds J. Palaganas, J. Maxworthy, C. Epps and M. Mancini), Wolters Kluwer, Philadelphia, PA, p. 607.

13 Bond, W.F., Lammers, R.L., Spillane, L.L. *et al.* (2007) The use of simulation in emergency medicine: a research agenda. *Acad Emerg Med*, **14** (4), 353–63. doi: 10.1197/j.aem.2006.11.021

14 Issenberg, S.B., Ringsted, C., Ostergaard, D. and Dieckmann, P. (2011) Setting a research agenda for simulation-based healthcare education: a synthesis of the outcome from an Utstein style meeting. *Simul Healthc*, **6** (3), 155–67. doi: 10.1097/SIH.0b013e3182207c24

15 Dieckmann, P., Phero, J.C., Issenberg, S.B. *et al.* (2011) The first Research Consensus Summit of the Society for Simulation in Healthcare: conduction and a synthesis of the results. *Simul Healthc.*, **6** (Suppl), S1–9. doi: 10.1097/SIH.0b013e31822238fc

16 Nestel, D., Groom, J., Eikeland-Husebo, S. and O'Donnell, J.M. (2011) Simulation for learning and teaching procedural skills: the state of the science. *Simul Healthc.*, **6** (Suppl), S10–13. doi: 10.1097/SIH.0b013e318227ce96

17 Raemer, D., Anderson, M., Cheng, A. *et al.* (2011) Research regarding debriefing as part of the learning process. *Simul Healthc*, **6** (7), S52–S7.

18 Kardong-Edgren, S., Gaba, D., Dieckmann, P. and Cook, D.A. (2011) Reporting inquiry in simulation. *Simul Healthc.*, **6** (Suppl), S63–6. doi: 10.1097/SIH.0b013e318228610a

19 Stefanidis, D., Arora, S., Parrack, D.M. *et al.* (2012) Research priorities in surgical simulation for the 21st century. *Am J Surg*, **203** (1), 49–53. doi: 10.1016/j.amjsurg.2011.05.008

20 Johnston, M.J., Paige, J.T., Aggarwal, R. *et al.* (2016) An overview of research priorities in surgical simulation: what the literature shows has been achieved during the 21st century and what remains. *Am J Surg*, **211** (1), 214–25. doi: 10.1016/j.amjsurg.2015.06.014

21 Nestel D, Watson M, Marshall S, Arora S, Bearman M. A national healthcare simulation research agenda: Process and outcomes. *Adv Simul. In review.*

22 INSPIRE. INSPIRE Network Report 2014–2015. 2015.

23 Simulation and Gaming [cited 22 November 2015]. Available from: http://sag.sagepub.com/

24 Simulation in Healthcare [cited 22 November 2015]. Available from: http://journals.lww.com/simulationinhealthcare/pages/default.aspx

25 Clinical Simulation in Nursing [cited 22 November 2015]. Available from: http://www.nursingsimulation.org/

26 BMJ Simulation and Technology Enhanced Learning [cited 22 November 2015]. Available from: http://stel.bmj.com/content/current

27 Advances in Simulation [cited 22 November 2015]. Available from: http://advancesinsimulation.biomedcentral.com/

28 Nestel, D. (2015) Expert's corner: funding for healthcare simulation research, in *Defining excellence in simulation programs* (eds J. Palaganas, J. Maxworthy, C. Epps and M. Mancini), Wolters Kluwer, Philadelphia, PA, p. 274.

CHAPTER 7

Simulated participant methodologies: Maintaining humanism in practice

Debra Nestel, Jill Sanko & Nancy McNaughton

KEY MESSAGES

- *Simulated participants* (SPs) are individuals who play the roles of others in scenarios – such as patients, clients, service users, healthcare professionals, students and so on [1].

- Specialized healthcare simulation practices have emerged such that those who work with SPs often do not work with confederates and so their methods have sometimes developed in isolation.

- There are points of intersection between simulated patients and confederate practices in simulation-based education, such as *emotional* work, which should be acknowledged in order to maintain humanism, a core underpinning of health professional education.

- Several strategies are offered that may strengthen SP role portrayal and feedback and mitigate any negative impact, and these require consideration before, during and after simulations.

Overview

This chapter explores the roles of simulated patients and confederates in simulation-based education. We use the collective term *simulated participant* (SP) for both and identify points of intersection in their work. A shared feature is the emotional component of their practice. This is an understudied area for SPs, especially for confederates. Educators have a responsibility to care for SPs; that is, to maintain humanism in simulation practices.

Introduction

In this chapter we explore the work of live 'simulators' in healthcare scenario-based simulations. There are two main types of live simulators. First, simulated (standardized) patients are individuals trained to portray a patient and also to provide feedback to trainees on their performance. Often, simulated patients are recruited from the community and may not necessarily have professional acting experience. Second, confederates are individuals who commonly portray the role of healthcare professionals in mannequin-based scenarios. They are usually recruited from local faculty, although there are many variations. What is notable is that simulated patients and confederates work with educators who often practise in isolation as a consequence of the locale of their primary simulation modality. That is, for simulated patient educators, their primary modality is simulated patients, while for educators who work with confederates, their primary modality is usually mannequins. In common is the critical addition of a human element to scenario-based simulations. With the recognition of the human element comes a responsibility for the humanity of those involved, simulated patients and confederates alike. Our focus in this chapter is to draw attention to these humanistic elements of simulation. Throughout the chapter we adopt the inclusive term *simulated participant* [1] when referring to simulated patients and confederates. Where we make reference to specific roles and experiences, we revert to simulated patient or confederate.

Simulated patients have a long history in healthcare simulations, with the first documented accounts based in the USA with the work of Howard Barrows in medical education [2]. Although now represented in the curricula of most health and social care professionals, the published literature is most commonly located in medical education. An important driver to development of the methodology has been the ubiquitous use of the objective structured clinical examination (OSCE). This summative assessment role has also influenced the focus on 'standardization'. That is, when simulated patients are required to produce the same performance consistently for participant learners, simulated patients effectively become the exam question, enabling each learner to be offered the *same* question [3]. However, simulated patients have also had a dominant role in formative assessment, where their individuality is valued. Nestel has also argued for valuing simulated patients as proxies for real patients, thereby foregrounding their re-presentation of patients rather than being agents for clinicians [4].

From a previous publication [5] comes the following description:

> Confederates usually play the role of a health or social care professional or a patient's relative and are often 'alone' in the scenario. That is, they are immersed in the scenario as an agent of the simulation educator or researcher as opposed to one of the participant group. They may also play the role of visitors, first responders (e.g. police, firemen) or witnesses (e.g. passerby at a motor vehicle accident). Confederates are most commonly colleagues (e.g. simulation educators, clinicians, research associates, etc.) or actors employed for this specific role. Sometimes participants other than the intended learner group are recruited as confederates, while in some simulations a fellow participant may be asked to take on this role.

Unlike simulated patient roles, confederate roles are often primarily developed as an agent for the educator. There are many commonalities in simulated patient and confederate work (Box 7.1). An important point of intersection is the emotional work in both roles. However, before shifting our focus to these emotional elements and offering considerations for educators in caring for SPs, we will explore the roles of simulated patients and confederates in more detail.

Box 7.1 Summary of the practices of simulated participants

Guide learners

- Orientate learners to the scenario
- Help learners work in an unfamiliar simulation environment
- Prompt learners at specified points – verbal and material/task
- Guide learners to meet learning objectives
- Offer feedback at pre-planned teachable moments, including the debriefing

Offer safety

- Provide physical safety for learners
- Protect simulators from damage/potential harm

Add realism

- Demonstrate appropriate emotions (e.g. sad, happy, cooperative, anxious and arrogant)
- Provide relevant cues to compensate in simulator fidelity (e.g. an infant's mother states 'he is so sleepy' or 'his hands are so cold!')
- Increase learners' engagement in the scenario by selectively increasing participants' cognitive load

Bridge between faculty and learners

- Respond to audio or other cues from faculty during scenarios
- Communicate with 'control room' during scenarios
- Offer insider experience during debriefing and/or evaluation

Provide assessments

- Use rating forms to make judgements on learners' performance

Facilitate research

- Observe actions and collect data not otherwise able to be collected unobtrusively (e.g. a nurse confederate would be able to observe a dose of medication prepared by a pharmacist prior to administration)
- Standardize the manner in which information is conveyed to study participants (e.g. laboratory data, physical signs and symptoms, whether the patient has a known allergy and so forth) to limit variability and minimize the risk of bias

Source: Adapted from Nestel et al, 2014.

Simulated patients work with health professional trainees and practitioners in a multiplicity of clinical formative and assessment activities. As proxies for patients they take on physical and emotional attributes, which they teach through their role portrayals and quite often also through their feedback following the simulation. Simulated patients use their bodies and minds to tell clinical stories – which are usually not their own. Engaging people in simulation requires educators to acknowledge the real possibility that the emotions (e.g. pain, grief, anxiety) in which we ask them to participate in the service of health professional trainees' and clinicians' learning may unintentionally be produced for real and therefore fully experienced and felt. Furthermore, simulated patients are often objectified by faculty, which may diminish their humanity and devalue their equality as co-teachers [6]. Anecdotes from simulated patients often describe simple acts by faculty that reduce their status, such as the location and quality of meeting rooms (e.g. far away from the examination area) and the food and refreshments offered to them compared with faculty examiners at OSCEs.

While confederates are also asked to engage in emotional work, the nature of this work may be different. Nestel et al. have documented that when confederates are faculty, especially junior colleagues or those asked to play caricatures (e.g. orthopaedic surgeons as autocratic, operating theatre nurses as clock watchers etc.), this can have a negative impact on them [5]. Aspiring surgical students invited to play roles as underperforming surgical trainees were concerned that the surgeons (learners in the simulations) may hold an enduring image of them as underperforming, unable to separate the confederates' identity from their real one. Additionally, experienced nurses have reported similar concerns when asked to play the role of unprofessional nurses, questioning the value of perpetuating unhelpful stereotypes. Like simulated patients, confederates asked to play the roles of simulated relatives may experience strong emotional reactions.

Caring for simulated participants

We have organized the remainder of the chapter into strategies to care for simulated participants across phases; that is, before, during and after simulations (Box 7.2). We acknowledge overlap with actions in later phases contingent on prior considerations. In each phase, we consider simulated patients prior to confederates. We also offer examples of scenarios with SPs to illustrate the strategies (Box 7.3).

Box 7.2 Strategies that educators can use to care for simulated participants

Before the simulation

Preparation

- Determine the considerations needed for appropriate recruitment and selection for roles (casting) of simulated participants
- Description of learning activity (and related logistics)
  a. Formative, summative
  b. Learning objectives/outcomes
  c. Length, frequency, rotations, repetitions
  d. Time outs
  e. Feedback, video-assisted debriefing – written, spoken, facilitated, timing
  f. Evaluation – written, spoken
  g. De-roling
- Descriptions of role, character, task
- Descriptions of learners, including their discipline, level, task, expected performance, prior experience, potential challenges
- Description of scenario, including the setting, length (and scenario-related logistics)
- Ensure proper attire is available and worn and consistent with the role (e.g. simulated patient wears 'abuse' blouse, simulated participant playing a surgeon wears scrubs)

Briefing

- Considerations include when, where, who (with/without learners, with/without faculty), how long, checking in, opportunity for further questions, indication of start, finish and time-out cues

During the simulation

- Direct/indirect observation of what is happening in the simulation, who is permitted to be present and who can observe, enactment of cues as briefed
- Direct/indirect observation of observers of the simulation, including maintenance of privacy, minimal talking, constructive use of rating forms
- Observation for potential safety issues and being poised to intervene to maintain the safety of the learners and/or simulated participants

After the simulation

- Facilitate de-roling of simulated participants by introducing them to learners by their real name (and where relevant role), moving to a different space to that of the simulation, conscious shedding of emotion/behaviour from scenario
- Provide support to simulated participants to offer frank and honest feedback in rating forms and/or during debriefing
- Seek feedback from simulated participants on their experiences of the simulation to inform quality improvements
- Encourage simulated patients to move about between scenarios, to stretch limbs (e.g. if holding in a particular position during the scenario), neck rolls, shoulder rolls, concentrate on breathing
- If simulated patients are playing emotionally demanding roles, then encourage them to plan something uplifting afterwards
- Remind simulated participants that emotionally demanding roles may affect them later and offer a follow-up contact
- Propose additional strategies to simulated participants such as writing a journal, meditation or other de-stressing activities the individual enjoys

Box 7.3 Examples of Simulated Participant Roles

Simulated patient in an OSCE for summative assessment

Albert Jones is a retired engineer and has been recruited to a university simulated patient program. He is invited to a training session where he will learn about the ways in which the medical school works with simulated patients to test their medical students' inpatient assessment tasks and physical examinations. The first 3-hour session introduces medical terms, assessment skills and exercises to portray patients realistically. Following participation in this session, Mr Jones will return prior to playing a patient to receive training specific to his role(s). This includes scenario briefing, specific role information, student expectations, assessment criteria of learners and session evaluation. On the day of the encounter Mr Jones will play the patient ten times and evaluate ten learners individually. He will also participate in debriefing with learners, providing feedback on their performance from the perspective of the patient. Following completion of his day, he will be given feedback regarding his own performance, assisted in stepping out of the role and paid for his time.

Confederate in a mock code scenario for formative assessment

Betty Jones is a nurse educator and uses simulation-based education to provide training to the nurses at the hospital in which she works. Each week the intensive care unit (ICU) nurses and physicians who respond to codes within the hospital participate in a mock code scenario. Today's scenario is depicting a patient who has severe respiratory distress secondary to a pulmonary embolism. A high-technology mannequin will represent the patient. Betty will be playing the confederate, a floor nurse who called a code for the patient because of worsening respiratory distress. The confederate (nurse) is nervous when the team (learners) show up to assess the patient. She is worried that the patient's distress is from something she did. Part of the objectives of the simulation include the confederate providing help and information about the patient, but the learners need to recognize and respond to her nervousness in order to access valuable information. Just prior to the scenario starting, Betty reviews the scenario, her role and the goals and objectives of the scenario. Her role is loosely scripted, but she feels comfortable ad-libbing as needed. Following the scenario, she will co-debrief with a physician educator. To facilitate the role change, her physician colleague will encourage her to de-role immediately after the scenario.

Simulated patients and confederates in a formative assessment

A large academic medical centre trains a number of residents each year. Because these new residents may not see every type of patient during training, the hospital uses simulation-based education to present low-volume high-risk patients. Today several residents will be participating in a scenario that involves a woman arriving in the emergency department for a broken arm secondary to domestic abuse. A simulated patient will be playing the patient role and one of the nurse educators from the simulation centre will be the confederate, a triage nurse who first encounters the patient. The simulated patient is from the university's simulated patient programme. The simulated patient received her scenario preparation and briefing earlier and is ready to go. There will be no assessment of the learners for this scenario. The confederate has read over the scenario, the script and the objectives. Both the simulated patient and the confederate will participate in debriefing. The simulated patient will participate in debriefing, along with the confederate as an educator. Following the scenario and debriefing encounters, the team will debrief, discussing aspects of the scenario in need of improvement as well as aspects that went well.

Before the simulation

Recruitment, screening and role portrayal training practices are important in making sure that simulated patients can work effectively and be protected against unintended emotional effects. Sometimes even the most *neutral*-seeming scenario can cause a simulated patient emotional or psychological trouble if it triggers a memory or experience. All simulated participants need to understand the parameters and context of the activity in which they will be engaged, so it is important to impart information such as the purpose of a scenario, how many times they may have to repeat it or how long they will remain in role, and whether they are responsible for completing a checklist/rating form or providing verbal feedback. This information allows them to understand the scope of their responsibilities and expectations and to prepare more fully for their roles.

Two key factors to consider when recruiting and preparing simulated patients are the proximity of the role to the simulated patient's own life circumstances relating to *role adherence* and the *role fit* [7]. With respect to 'role adherence', it can be harder for a simulated patient to shed a role if the scenario is too close to their own life or written in such a way that they need to call on their own history and personal details for information. The particulars of the character's condition (physical, psychological, social and economic) or complaint may stick to the simulated patient like invisible threads that are difficult to remove. So it is important during recruitment and training activities to be transparent about role portrayal expectations. Simulated patients must be made aware that they should notify someone at any point in the training or work process if they feel uncomfortable. Additionally, if, during the training or another point in their work as a simulated patient, an individual feels uncomfortable or appears to be having trouble with the role, there should be a mechanism for a follow-up conversation, the option to withdraw and additional resources offered (e.g. psychological help).

The concept of 'role fit' refers to simulated patients who are too close to or too far from the temperament, personality or experience of the person they will be portraying. Uncomfortable feelings may be evoked in the simulated patient by the role play for reasons unrelated to the simulation. For example, many people are uncomfortable displaying anger. This is not due to any

specific situation, but is difficult for their temperament or personality. The opposite can also be problematic. A key variable in the fit between the role and the simulated patient is their psychological sophistication or ability to understand their own personal make-up. Recruiting the right simulated patient for a nuanced psychological portrayal may require that they have the ability to differentiate between themselves and the role even though there may be similarities. From a study conducted by Woodward, a simulated patient stated: 'The thing is that through it all [role playing] it is touching things in me and bringing things out in me I wouldn't have been aware of before' [8]. The simulated patient needs to understand clearly the fit between them and the role that they are playing in order to avoid uncomfortable reactions both during and following role enactment. Woodward reported that some simulated patients chose to stop playing disturbing roles (incest survivor, alcoholic, schizophrenic or rape victim) that they had played previously because they found themselves feeling unsettled [8].

With a few exceptions, there is little empirically based published work on the recruitment and preparation of confederates for scenarios. Sanko et al. [9] and Nestel et al. [5] offer theory- and experience-based accounts of supporting confederates. Sanko et al. draw from the discipline of acting to provide guidance in refining the practice of simulation by embracing lessons and techniques commonly used in the theatre (performing arts) community, while Nestel et al. highlight the importance of drawing on practices from simulated patient methodology for character development and role portrayal.

During the simulation

Simulated patient work is not therapy, educators are not therapists and we are not suggesting that the details of simulated patients' personal stories even need to be known. However, it is important to support simulated patients in their experience with a role. In a study exploring the effects of emotionally complex roles, simulated patients reported that there were roles that they would never do again because of the similarity between the role and their own life [7]. Personal discomfort with an aspect of a role may inhibit simulated patients from responding in a way that is clinically accurate, appropriate or correctly portrayed. It is therefore important for the quality of the educational session that those portraying the roles can do so to the required level of realism and accuracy. For the same reason, if a simulated patient is struggling with an affect or physical aspect of a role, they need to be supported in their decision to discontinue involvement. It may be that at this time the simulated patient is experiencing something in their own life that prevents them from taking part. However, at a later time they may be fine. This kind of attention to the simulated patient's well-being also has implications for their employment retention. Acknowledging that simulated patient work is not meant to cause harm to those who are portraying roles for educational purposes recognizes the humanity of the SP. In the end, a fully developed character that is different enough in personal and clinical history from the simulated patient may in fact prove to be a mitigating factor in emotional fallout or role adherence. For, although a character and a simulated patient may share many of the same emotional, psychological and physical features, the boundary between the life stories makes it easier for the simulated patient to move back into their real life. For the confederate, simulating one's own role can raise questions of self-doubt in a way similar to the boundary blurring just discussed. It is therefore as important if not more so for people in a confederate role to acknowledge the differences between their performance in the role and in their everyday practice.

Training techniques can be used to help simulated participants take on a role while also clearly separating themselves from the role. However, there are instances in which there is no time or opportunity for a simulated participant to learn a role and practise it over time.

Information about what to do to keep SPs safe and fresh during or after a simulation should be sought, respected and acted on.

After the simulation

De-roling

With respect to shedding or stepping out of a role, sometimes called de-roling, actors are likely to be more familiar with techniques of transition than non-actors. They may be more likely to think of the simulation as an acting job and as a result be able to maintain a clear distinction between themselves and the role

they are playing. They are also more likely to have techniques that they use to shed a role, such as the activity of taking off make-up or sometimes putting on make-up to return to the day-to-day world. Some simulated patients have particular clothes that they reserve for different, more emotionally challenging roles. An experienced simulated patient reported to one of the authors that she has an 'abuse' blouse that she never wears unless doing the role. When she takes it off, it is an important indicator of her return to her life. Another simulated patient always calls a family member on her way home from work as a way of checking back in or resuming *her* life. Other such techniques for returning to self are often shared between simulated patients who are doing the same role, such as simple mindful meditation before and after simulations and consciously acknowledging that this work may be difficult. For simulated patients it is important to recognize that psychological and emotional distress is not always felt during or immediately following a simulation, but may take time to filter through and be felt. It is not unusual for simulated patients to report lingering effects even days later. Writing a journal is a good way to decompress, process events and separate the simulation experience from one's own life. It is important for educators engaging simulated patients in difficult emotional simulations to hear about their experiences. Arranging a time to check in several days after a simulation session is helpful.

The physical effects of crying all day, sometimes every ten minutes during an OSCE, or having to revisit an angry or manipulative affect may require physical activity to break the role adherence. One author (NM) reports that following a day of portraying a person with antisocial personality disorder in an OSCE, a simulated patient felt so angry when driving home that he had to pull over and rest before continuing [10]. He reported that he went for a run as soon as he got home and felt much better afterwards. This response was only identified a week later despite the team having 'touched base' with him following the exam.

A simple technique includes having the simulated participant introduce themselves to learners by their real name, explicitly shedding the emotion and behaviours they were portraying in the scenario and adopting their usual persona following an interaction. This gives an immediate opportunity for all to recalibrate to one another's real-life roles and close the door on the prior encounter. Moving the debriefing session to a space different to that in which the simulation occurred is also helpful. Whether simulated participants are involved in the debriefing usually needs to be planned ahead of time. If they are not included, then learners may need to be reminded that simulated participants were playing roles. The amount of information shared with learners about the simulated participants would be negotiated with them, but usually does not involve much information. For example, 'the simulated patients you worked with today are part of the programme here at the university' or 'the confederate in the scenario is a simulation fellow in anaesthesia who has just joined our team. Her portrayal of the operating theatre nurse does not reflect her usual practice'.

Debriefing with learners

SPs are often required to share their experiences with learners during debriefings. SPs are usually asked to step out of role to offer feedback, as already outlined. There are few circumstances where it is helpful to stay in role. The debriefing may be facilitated by educators or SPs or may be learner led. During debriefing, learners' emotions are often aroused, sometimes with disappointment about their performance and with a sense of foreboding about what the debriefing may uncover. SPs may also be experiencing strong emotions about learners' helpful and unhelpful behaviours. An SP must feel psychologically safe to share their experiences with the learners. Offering constructive feedback on unhelpful behaviours is especially challenging. SPs usually require training to support development of the content and language of feedback and debriefing processes. Acknowledging to all those participating in the debriefing that being in the scenario often feels utterly different to being an observer can be a first step to validating statements about the interaction and its effects on the SP. It is also acceptable for SPs to hold different views to educators and to learners and these differences need to be respected. Facilitators have an important role here in making this explicit.

Evaluation of the simulation and debriefing the simulated participants

The term 'evaluation' here refers to the success of the simulation in meeting the needs of the learners. Quality improvement may include discussion with the simulated participants of the usefulness of written materials

used in preparation, training for role portrayal, the rating form, debriefing with learners and commentary on the learners' performances. Evaluation may focus on what was easy and what was hard in the scenario, from the simulated participants' perspective. The overall goal is to improve the preparation and implementation of the learning session. Discussing the impact of learners' behaviours on role portrayal is important for potential modification of the role for future sessions. This is also an opportunity to provide simulated participants with feedback on role portrayal and their feedback to learners. Principles of effective feedback need to be modelled during this process to reinforce considerate educational methods.

The format for debriefing the SPs will vary depending on the related simulation activities. For example, in an OSCE, a simulated patient debriefing is likely to be in a large group. However, the quality improvement elements of a debriefing could also be collected in an evaluation form. Confederates are usually fewer in number and as such the format may be one to one or in a small group with other faculty. There is a danger that the emotional work of confederates in simulation activities may be forgotten, for a number of reasons. There may be a small number of confederates, the single person and the task are simply overlooked or perhaps incorrect assumptions are made about their identity and coping strategies. Of equal importance, the confederate may be a healthcare colleague. This is very important to acknowledge, especially if they have been asked to perform in the simulation scenario in a way and to a standard different to their usual professional role.

In the context of simulated patients, the value of debriefing is variable, although further research is required to better understand the consequences for simulated patients of this work. Some simulated patients have reported that they resent having to attend debriefing sessions, while other simulated patients report depending on them. Simulated patients who took part in focus groups following a psychiatry OSCE reported needing to retreat into themselves for a few days and to treat themselves almost as if they had been sick, taking long baths and not engaging too vigorously in social or physical activity. As one SP noted: 'If I don't sufficiently acknowledge that my psyche has visited a very vulnerable place, it will come back to haunt me three or four days later as deep fatigue' [7].

experience being enacted in real time. A crucial feature is that it is *neurobiologically subjective*, reeling in the individual's sense making and presence into the story building. It captures forms of meaning making that go beyond the technical and procedural to incorporate the sensory and emotive elements that also have impacts on clinical decision making.

We can track how the macro narrative and the neurobiological (subjective) micro narrative sense-making processes collide to provide a more complex picture of the totality of internal perception, situation awareness and decision making in expert clinicians.

The pilot study

Macro and micro dramaturgy

To examine this dramaturgical sense-making paradigm within simulation, we set up a re-enactment of an emergency crisis scenario. Four anaesthetists – all highly experienced consultants – were put through a real-time emergency crisis. The deliberate focus on experts put the spotlight on complex decision making rather than procedural learning, as might have been the case in simulation training for novices. The RAH had never conducted simulation exercises with experienced clinicians, and this was a way of piloting the merits of a programme aimed at reviewing high-level clinical and decision-making skills.

Our dramaturgical approach was to centre specifically on the 'explicit' macro narrative and the 'implicit' subjective micro narratives extracted from and during the enactment. While acknowledging that medical simulation is a team process, the study deliberately focused on the macro and micro levels in order to explore how the expert or clinician was constructing meaning from the enactment. This is the, often neglected, phenomenological component of consultant sense making.

Undeniably the greatest challenge for the study was the elicitation of the micro narrative as a direct, first-person lived experience. The macro narrative was readily accessible in terms of the clinical scenario and plan put forward by the simulation director. However, there was no clear methodology to access the experiential micro narrative. Existing conventions for non-technical briefing and video recording that allowed participants to view and review their behaviour did not appear to tap deeply enough into the subject's

internal sense making. Debriefing methodologies are a significant aspect of healthcare simulation practice, with a range of frameworks currently being discussed within the field [4]. In the study our focus was not so much on the debriefing process per se, but on how to capture the raw, subjective moment-by-moment experience of the clinicians and their neurobiological subjective processing.

Given the interdisciplinary nature of the collaboration, we adopted an experimental aggregation of techniques drawn from verbatim theatre, a form of documentary theatre that draws on real-life testimonies, the naturalistic decision making (NDM) or subjective recall methods fostered by Gary Klein [5] and experimental neurophenomenological protocols first established by neuroscientist Francesco Varela to elicit a spontaneous evocation of the lived experience. Varela's protocols in particular cemented our phenomenological strategy [6].

The narrative and dramaturgical analysis

The macro narrative for the pilot can be summarized as follows:

> A young man who has suffered a car accident is lying bleeding on an operating table. During the course of the treatment the accident victim is given doses of gelofusine (a version of saline solution) and he has an allergic reaction, which causes further deterioration and leads to anaphylaxis.

It is a story fixed across time. In the words of the simulation director (see also Box 8.1):

> I am just trying to keep a story running: once it is up and running I am not changing the scenario, just marrying things that happen with the path of the scenario.

Box 8.1 Anaphylaxis to gelofusine: Clinical scenario by Dr Graham Lowry

---

Time: 22.00 hrs setting: city hospital and trauma centre

Background history
An anaesthetic registrar on night duty has been asked to anaesthetize a 27-year-old male who has been involved in a motor vehicle accident. The patient was a front-seat passenger of a car that left the road and collided with a tree. The point of impact was on the driver's side, and the driver has sustained life-threatening chest injuries.

The patient, who was the passenger, had a GCS (Glasgow Coma Score) of 15/15 at the scene of the accident and was transferred to the hospital by ambulance. On arrival at hospital his observations were GCS 15/15, BP (blood pressure) 110/60, HR (heart rate) 95, SpO_2 (oxygen saturation) 98% on 6 L/min O_2. Initially he responded well to 2 L intravenous crystalloid fluid (normal saline), but his blood pressure then started to trend downwards.

Other relevant medical history
Part medical history: nil significant; medications: nil regular; allergies: none known; smoker: 15–20 cigs/day.

Clinical examination showed
Deformed right wrist – backslab plaster applied; seat-belt bruising left chest; tender abdomen; tender neck – spinal precautions taken according to trauma guidelines.

Investigations performed on arrival to the emergency department
C-spine X-ray: no abnormality detected (NAD); CXR (chest X-ray): NAD; X-ray pelvis: NAD; X-match blood: 4 units of packed red cells ordered; CT (computed tomography) abdomen: free fluid detected.

Within this metanarrative framework, the micro narrative traces the learner's subjective journey. As such, the micro narrative takes a non-linear, first-person perspective shaped by the moment-to-moment responses of the clinician's *bottom-up*, intuitive sensorimotor perceptions, together with their *top-down*, higher-level reflective functions. In essence, it is how they are perceiving the plot, as it unfolds to them. It offers a transient flow of sense making and sense giving, catching meanings as they materialize. Felt from within, it exists in a perpetual state of *presentness* as the consultants adjust to each new event and changing circumstance. The micro narratives and the consultants' journeys therefore stand as a form of embodied performance [7].

The excerpts in this section are extracts from verbatim consultant interviews and transcripts conducted between April and June 2011 as part of a doctoral investigation into narrative sense making in live simulation. The identity of the consultants has been deliberately kept anonymous. For complete transcripts and more detailed analysis see Crea [8]. The excerpts highlight perhaps the most salient features to emerge from our analysis. In particular, they underscore the fluid nature of real-time medical sense making and the degree to which it is shaped by non-linear, emotive and even at

times unpredictable responses. While the metanarrative is clear, linear and logical, the micro narrative is filled with ambiguity, uncertainty and emotion. Subjective narrative and story building do not unfold according to a linear, sequential paradigm. Meaning shifts with unfolding circumstances and underscores the dynamic nature of medical diagnosis. Consider this extract highlighting the tension between what exists externally and what the consultant is feeling internally:

I am quite sure that I can't hear air … I still can't believe there is air on the right hand side despite the nurse telling me there is air on both sides I couldn't hear it … I have made a diagnosis and the symptoms don't match … there was a conflict between the algorithm and the feedback.

The sense making is exposed to a complex system of interactions and sensations constantly adjusting in time:

I have made a diagnosis. Blood pressure is falling but I can't quite hear. In my mind, the diagnosis is not clear. Start to get anxious. Focus more on the heart. Beginning to believe there is another problem. Look at other possible causes of blood loss and hypertension. What on earth is going on with this patient? Where is this leading?

In confirming our proposal of simulation as an action narrative (drama), it is also clear that taking action is what propels the meaning making forward at the micro level. Meaning may start as a sensation, but it is given expression through what is actionable. Essentially, the consultants move from one action response to another.

my focus (emphasis) was shifting between the monitors and the patient, glancing at the monitors to look at what the situation was, then focus on the patient thinking through what action I needed to take … in a situation where things weren't clear I needed to move and the way to move was to take action …

Need to move on. Need to take action. Act and sort. You need to get in to make it happen.

The narrative sense making is clearly enacted, emerging from the interplay of action and perception.

It is also obvious that narrative meaning encapsulates a subjective mix of attention, sensory perception, pattern recognition, memory and personal history. All of the consultants highlight anxiety at needing to work through ambiguity, confusion and uncertainty, and how

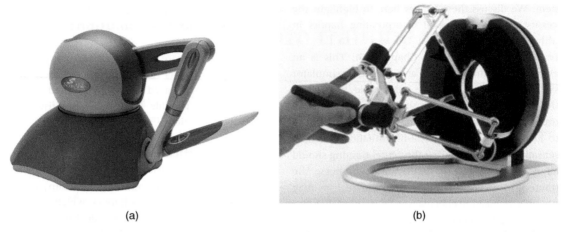

(a)   (b)

Figure 9.1 Examples of existing single-point desktop kinaesthetic haptic devices: (a) Phantom Omni from Geomagic (formerly Sensable); (b) Omega 6 from Force Dimension.

applicable to these devices include minimal invasive surgery, endoscopy and orthopaedic surgery (arthroscopy and trauma surgery).

- Multifinger haptic devices (usually between 2 and 5 fingers) are intended for healthcare training simulations where interfinger operations such as pinch, grasp and injection are highly regarded [7–9]. These devices usually omit dual-hand operations and are best suited for healthcare procedures focusing on single-hand operations, such as foreign body removal, epidural injection and lumbar puncture. Although some of these training scenarios actually require both hands to finish, many existing device set-ups focus only on the part where the main force feedback is rendered.

- Holistic haptic devices are more sophisticated configurations that are capable of providing both kinaesthetic and tactile feedback simultaneously. They can be significantly more useful in procedures requiring both kinaesthetic and tactile feedback, such as training simulation of a complex healthcare procedure involving palpation, injection, incision and suturing. One major challenge for holistic haptic devices is to identify the proper approach to integrate both types of feedback in the HIPs and associating the tactile feedback devices (usually an array of vibrators or pins) with the transformation of their corresponding HIPs.

Although research on these advanced haptic devices has been progressing, many projects are still at the prototype stage. With the growth of more accurate and capable haptic devices, the quality of healthcare training simulation systems is expected to be further improved.

Application examples

Since the early days of haptics research, healthcare training simulation has been one of the key application domains. Over the years, a number of haptics-driven healthcare training systems have been proposed, implemented and validated from both industrial and research facilities.

The key areas of existing haptics-driven healthcare training simulators are as follows:

- Minimal invasive surgery simulator systems, such as the insight ARTHRO VR [10] from GMV; the prototype system described in Nudehi et al. [11]; Laerdal's Virtual IV system [12], an intravenous catheterization learning and training system in IV insertion and phlebotomy; and the ImmersiveTouch [13], a training simulator for open and percutaneous surgeries. In addition, there are also a number of laparoscopic surgery simulator systems available [14–16].

- Endoscopic training simulator systems, such as the EndoscopyVR system [17] for gastrointestinal surgery and bronchoscopy; and the MicroVisTouch system [18] for microsurgery procedures such as endoscopic neurosurgery.

- Epidural injection simulator systems, such as the Yantric EpiSim system [19]; the Mediseus Epidural system [20] from Medic Vision; and the work described in Dang et al. [21].

- Orthopaedic training simulator systems, such as the TraumaVision system [22] from Melerit Medical AB; the MAKO RIO [23] system from Immersion; and the lumbar puncture simulator system described in Gorman et al. [24].
- Dental training simulators, such as the Individual Dental Education Assistant [25] from IDEA International; and the Simodont Dental Trainer system [26] from Moog.

In recent years there has been new research effort in promoting healthcare training simulator systems. Some work focuses on the rendering and interaction algorithms for rigid (such as bone) and deformable (such as soft tissue) 3D models, while other work is more on specific medical training applications. We discuss this research in the following sections.

SimOptiX

A recent effort to push the limit of haptics-driven healthcare training simulator systems is the SimOptiX project, a haptically enabled optometry training simulator that features not only interactive training simulation using haptics, but also seamless integration with an actual slit lamp that optometrists and ophthalmologists use on a daily basis.

The simulator has undergone two major stages, with two distinct hardware configurations targeting trainees with different training requirements.

The first configuration is based on haptics with head mount display (HMD) and augmented reality (AR). It is targeted at optometry students, who mostly focus on isolated and repetitive training simulation sessions. The system consists of both visual and haptic pipelines, which run in parallel. In the haptic rendering pipeline, a standard Phantom Omni device is mounted next to the slit lamp, with careful hardware calibration on its location and rotation. In the visual rendering pipeline, a webcam captures the position and rotation of AR markers located on the eyes of a dummy head and visualizes the anatomy of a virtual eye through the HMD. All haptic-related operations will also be visualized during the training session. A number of key parameters for the immersive and accurate simulation of various optometry procedures have also been implemented in the configuration, such as the angle, distance and brightness of the head light, needle sharpness, eye

separations for stereo vision and so on. Two typical training scenarios have been identified and implemented, including the needle-injection procedure and the foreign body–removal procedure. Different force-rendering algorithms have also been implemented to support the distinctive force variations during the procedures due to different tool choices. A small scale user study was conducted and most participants are positive about the accuracy and immersion of this configuration [27].

The second configuration is targeted at established optometrists and ophthalmologists to maintain and improve their procedural skills. This configuration is heavily involved with various absolute measurement sensors, which are electronically integrated into the slit lamp and replace many of its original optical pathway components. The integrated sensors are connected to the original control parts on the slit lamp and seamlessly translate user input into digital signals, which are reflected through multipoint haptic devices and visual rendering results. The detailed control layout is illustrated in Figure 9.2, and the actual system in action is demonstrated in Figure 9.3. Two rendering algorithms based on texture blending and masking as well as shading language were implemented [28], and their rendering results were compared to justify the visual immersions.

Based on this configuration, another user study has been conducted to validate its practicability as well as its comparative impressions with the first configuration. Results showed that a more natural user interaction interface, which in this case is the standard layout of control components on a slit lamp, could further improve the success rate and the immersion of the training simulation [29].

SimNeT

SimNeT is a haptics-driven needle thoracostomy training simulator system for tension pneumothorax, which is an emergency condition where excessive air accumulates in the pleural cavity following a lung or airway injury and exerts pressure on the lung, forcing it to collapse, as well as restricting cardiac output. Needle thoracostomy helps remove the air from the pleural cavity and prevents cardiac and respiratory failure. The key procedures of a needle thoracostomy are:

- Identify correct intercostal spaces through palpation.
- Identify different body components with distinct physical properties before needle introduction; that is, ribs are rigid while skin and lungs are deformable.

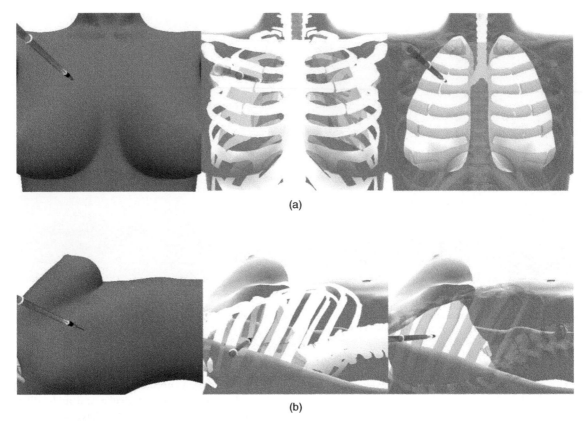

Figure 9.5 (a) X-ray view of multiple layered organs and tissues of pleural cavity for assisting trainees in validating haptic feedback with the actual organ/tissue touched. (b) Both mid-clavicular and mid-axillary approaches are shown.

incision force with every slight movement during the incision procedure. The identified and adjustable key parameters for the training simulator include:

- Tissue properties, such as skin elasticity and layered components under the skin.
- Scalpel properties, such as sharpness, blade shape and bevel angle.
- Operational properties, such as the velocity of the incision, and the magnitude and direction of the forces applied to the tissue.

Although incisions are usually short strokes, curved incisions are used in surgical procedures such as excision of skin lesions. To simulate such procedures, a curve-simplification algorithm has been proposed to convert continuous curves into three categories of grid-based split-line segments (horizontal, vertical and diagonal), which then splits the underlying deformation model accordingly and simulates the actual incision. Figure 9.6 is an initial demonstration of the interactive

incision simulation (halfway and full-length incision), while Figure 9.7 illustrates the curve-simplification algorithm. Note that the actual simplification algorithm involves higher resolution of the grids and the simplified incision segments are much closer to the incision curve.

SimInc is targeted at the performance and result analysis of human-centred incision simulations. On the other hand, robotic surgery has been rapidly evolving during the past decades, and this focuses on the consistency of surgery performance and the reduction of human involvement during surgery. They may seem to contradict each other, but they are actually heading towards the same goal from different perspectives. Eventually, it is humans who design and implement algorithms for robotic surgeries, and there will always be unpredictable cases with which robotic surgery may not cope. In the future, human-centred surgical training may not be as important as it is now, but simulation training tools can always keep surgeons' skills up to

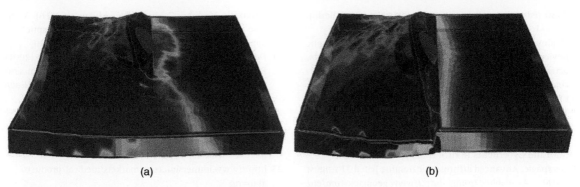

(a)   (b)

Figure 9.6 Different incisions based on the user's stroke through a soft body.

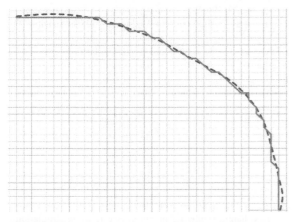

Figure 9.7 The interactive curve-simplification algorithm to render the user's stroke in grid-based segments. The actual simplification algorithm involves higher resolution of the grids and the simplified incision segments are much closer to the incision curve.

date and enable them to deal with difficult cases when necessary.

Conclusion and future work

Haptics-driven healthcare training simulations have been replacing traditional training simulations in the second decade of the twenty-first century, and this trend is still growing. The immersion of haptics into training content and its effectiveness in training results have helped healthcare professionals in a number of challenging scenarios. With the further development of hardware (especially multipoint haptics) and software (cross-vendor, extensible kinaesthetic and tactile communication frameworks), haptics is expected to play a more essential role in the healthcare sector. As patient-based training exposure becomes scarce, society still expects practitioners to become increasingly skilled. Haptics simulation modules allow healthcare students to gain valuable experience in a safe setting, while not putting patients at risk, thus helping to improve the quality of healthcare to the community.

References

1 Kammermeier, P., Kron, A., Hoogen, J. and Schmidt, G. (2004) Display of holistic haptic sensations by combined tactile and kinesthetic feedback. *Presence: Teleoper Virtual Environ.*, **13**, 1–15.

2 Minamizawa, K., Prattichizzo, D. and Tachi, S. (2010) Simplified design of haptic display by extending one-point kinesthetic feedback to multipoint tactile feedback, in *Haptics Symposium*, IEEE, pp. 257–60.

3 Fritschi M, Ernst MO, Buss M. (2006) Integration of kinesthetic and tactile display: a modular design concept. In: *Proceedings of the EuroHaptics 2006 International Conference*. The Eurohaptics Society: Paris, pp. 607–12.

4 Loi-Wah, S., Van Meer, F., Bailly, Y. and Chung Kwong, Y. (2007) Design and development of a Da Vinci surgical system simulator, in *International Conference on Mechatronics and Automation*, IEEE, pp. 1050–55.

5 Ullrich, S. and Kuhlen, T. (2012) Haptic palpation for medical simulation in virtual environments. *IEEE Trans Vis Comput Graph.*, **18**, 617–25.

6 Peer, A. and Buss, M. (2008) A new admittance-type haptic interface for bimanual manipulations. *IEEE/ASME Trans Mechatronics.*, **13**, 416–28.

7 Wei, L., Sourin, A., Najdovski, Z. and Nahavandi, S. (2012) Function-based single and dual point haptic interaction in cyberworlds, in *Transactions on computational science XVI*, vol.

7380 (eds M. Gavrilova and C.J.K. Tan), Springer, Berlin, pp. 1–16.

8 Najdovski, Z. and Nahavandi, S. (2008) Extending haptic device capability for 3D virtual grasping, in *Haptics: perception, devices and scenarios. Proceedings of the 6th international conference, Madrid, Spain*, vol. **5024** (ed. M. Ferre), Springer, Berlin, pp. 494–503.

9 Wei L, Najdovski Z, Hailing Z, Deshpande S, Nahavandi S. Extending support to customised multi-point haptic devices in CHAI3D. In: *2014 IEEE International Conference on Systems*, Man and Cybernetics (SMC). IEEE, pp. 1864–7.

10 Geomagic. Advanced arthroscopic training [cited 31 August 2016]. Available from: http://www.geomagic.com/en/products/haptic-applications/haptic-application-gallery/insight-arthro/

11 Nudehi, S.S., R. , Mukherjee, R. and Ghodoussi, M. (2005) A shared-control approach to haptic interface design for minimally invasive telesurgical training. *IEEE Trans Contr Syst Technol.*, **13**, 588–92.

12 http://www.immersion.com/markets/medical/products/#tab=viv

13 ImmersiveTouch. Simulators ImmersiveTouch® [cited 31 August 2016]. Available at: http://www.immersivetouch.com/ImmersiveTouch.html

14 Basdogan, C., Ho, C.H. and Srinivasan, M.A. (2001) Virtual environments for medical training: graphical and haptic simulation of laparoscopic common bile duct exploration. *IEEE/ASME Trans Mechatronics.*, **6**, 269–85.

15 Panait, L., Akkary, E., Bell, R.L. *et al.* (2009) The role of haptic feedback in laparoscopic simulation training. *J Surg Res.*, **156**, 312–16.

16 Basdogan, C., Ho, C.H., Srinivasan, M.A. *et al.* (1998) Force interactions in laparoscopic simulations: haptic rendering of soft tissues. *Stud Health Technol Inform.*, **50**, 385–91.

17 http://www.immersion.com/markets/medical/products/#tab=cae-endo

18 Immersive Touch. Simulators Microvistouch® [cited 31 August 2016]. Available at: http://www.immersivetouch.com/Microvistouch.html

19 Yantric [cited 31 August 2016]. Available at: http://www.yantric.com/products.html

20 Geomagic. Mediseus Epidural [cited 31 August 2016]. Available at: http://www.geomagic.com/en/products/haptic-applications/haptic-application-gallery/medic-vision/

21 Dang, T., Annaswamy, T.M. and Srinivasan, M.A. (2001) Development and evaluation of an epidural injection simulator with force feedback for medical training. *Stud Health Technol Inform.*, **81**, 97–102.

22 Geomagic. Melerit Medical – Trauma Vision [cited 31 August 2016]. Available at: http://www.geomagic.com/en/products/haptic-applications/haptic-application-gallery/melerit-medical/

23 http://www.immersion.com/markets/medical/products/#tab=rio

24 Gorman, P., Krummel, T., Webster, R. *et al.* (2000) A prototype haptic lumbar puncture simulator. *Stud Health Technol Inform.*, **70**, 106–9.

25 Geomagic. Individual Dental Education Assistant [cited 31 August 2016]. Available at: http://www.geomagic.com/en/products/haptic-applications/haptic-application-gallery/idea/

26 Moog. Haptic technology in the Moog Simodent dental trainer [cited 31 August 2016]. Available at: http://www.moog.com/markets/medical-dental-simulation/haptic-technology-in-the-moog-simodont-dental-trainer/

27 Wei L, Najdovski Z, Abdelrahman W, Nahavandi S, Weisinger H. Augmented optometry training simulator with multi-point haptics. In: *2012 IEEE International Conference on Systems*, Man, and Cybernetics (SMC). IEEE, pp. 2991–7.

28 Wei L, Huynh L, Zhou H, Nahavandi S. Immersive visuo-haptic rendering in optometry training simulation. *Paper presented at the 2014 IEEE International Conference on Systems*, Man and Cybernetics (SMC).

29 Wei, L., Najdovski, Z., Nahavandi, S. and Weisinger, H. (2014) Towards a haptically enabled optometry training simulator. *Netw Model Anal Health Inform Bioinform.*, **3**, 1–8.

30 Force Dimension. CHA13D [cited 31 August 2016]. Available at: http://www.forcedimension.com/products/chai3d/overview

CHAPTER 10

Virtual environments and virtual patients in healthcare

LeRoy Heinrichs, Parvati Dev & Dick Davies

KEY MESSAGES

- This chapter shows how virtual environments are being and could be developed and deployed in healthcare.

- A virtual environment (VE) is a real time, synchronous, persistent network of people, represented by avatars, facilitated by networked computers.

- VEs prepare students for clinical encounters so that time spent with patients is a safer and more valuable experience.

- When choosing a virtual world, the key criteria to consider are its accessibility, genre, adaptability and privacy.

- Interactive virtual patients are computer-based avatars exhibiting real-time normal or pathological signs and symptoms and often also treatable in real-time.

- Virtual patients offer the opportunity to create and deliver experiences that teach critical thinking, diagnostic reasoning and even communication.

- Barriers to the use of virtual environments in higher education include technology issues; student issues; institutional issues; and personal perceptions.

Overview

This chapter shows how 'virtualization technologies' are being developed and deployed in healthcare. First, it defines virtual environments and virtual patient technologies. Thereafter some examples of their uses in healthcare will be described. Interactive virtual patients are computer-based avatars exhibiting real-time normal or pathological signs and symptoms and often also treatable in real-time. The rationale for the deployment of these emerging technologies will then be addressed, before finally asking where virtual environments and virtual patients might be heading in tomorrow's healthcare environment.

Introduction

The junior doctor walks into the ward with a clinical colleague and asks to be directed to Mrs Fernandez, a recently admitted patient with sepsis. A ward nurse had called her to say that the patient had developed a red rash. The doctor introduces herself and her colleague to the patient and asks Mrs Fernandez how she is today. She checks the patient's medical record and then examines her with her colleague. Mrs Fernandez is uncomfortable, with a deep red rash. At this stage the doctor decides to involve a senior physician, who arrives and after discussion calls the pharmacist down to the ward to discuss the drug regime for the patient. The pharmacist reports that reactions can occur to some of the drugs administered. The senior physician diagnoses 'Red Man' syndrome on the basis of the pharmaceutical information. Treatment was prescribed and on follow-up the patient responded as expected, with the rash diminishing.

Real or virtual? In this case it was *both*, as this was a team interprofessional education (IPE) training exercise run at the Charles R. Drew/UCLA School of Medicine [1]. The student doctor entered the ward in a virtual hospital via her computer as an avatar. She then communicated in real time via her microphone and headset with her numerous clinical colleagues and the 'virtual patient', who were also in the virtual hospital as avatars. The dynamic 'virtual patient' responded as expected during her 'examination', demonstrating visually the signs of 'Red Man' syndrome, which in turn was linked

Healthcare Simulation Education: Evidence, Theory and Practice, First Edition.
Edited by Debra Nestel, Michelle Kelly, Brian Jolly and Marcus Watson.
© 2018 John Wiley & Sons Ltd. Published 2018 by John Wiley & Sons Ltd.

to the drugs administered as recorded in the electronic medical record and diagnosed following discussion with the pharmacist. The scenario reflects a medical error in that the rate of vancomycin administration was too rapid. (There is more on this case in Box 10.1.)

Unsurprisingly, these virtualization technologies are in day-to-day use in the recreational sector by many 'millennials' who are training to become tomorrow's healthcare professionals. This chapter shows how such

Box 10.1 Team interprofessional education

> Charles Drew University School of Medicine, an affiliate of University of California Los Angeles (UCLA), implemented a virtual environment with interactive virtual patients, the CliniSpace Virtual Sim Center (Permission given by IIL and Drew/UCLA for figure 10.1), to teach team-based interprofessional education. In a study of 60 students, the large majority, 90% or greater, reported ease of use, and 70% reported effective learning among team members about antibiotic overdose, due to the virtual patient avatars in an infection scenario developing a skin rash unique to excessive drugs use. The virtual rash subsided and the skin colour of the avatar returned to normal after the excessive rate of administration was corrected [1].

technologies are being developed and deployed in healthcare. First, it defines virtual environments and

virtual patient technologies. Thereafter some examples of their uses in healthcare are explored. The rationale for deployment will then be addressed, before finally asking where virtual environments and virtual patients might be heading in today's and tomorrow's healthcare.

Virtual environments and virtual patients

Virtual environments or virtual worlds are well-known technologies that were initially developed for recreational use by the computer gaming industry. They are now well-understood, stable technologies with many serious deployments in areas other than gaming, including retail, disaster response, procedure training in oil and gas, and marketing. On the other hand, virtual patients, while developed in the healthcare space, use a mixed range of media from patient actors, through paper exercises to computer-generated simulated patients.

What are virtual environments?

Also known as virtual worlds (VW), a virtual environment (VE) can be defined as a 'synchronous, persistent network of people, represented by avatars, facilitated by networked computers' [2]. Furthermore, 'a virtual

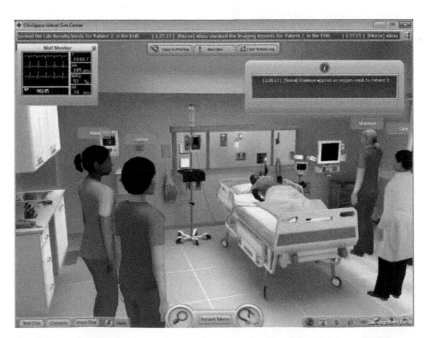

Figure 10.1 Learners in CliniSpace cooperating in treating a patient. Source: Copyright IIL & Drew/UCLA.

world operates in real time, exists whether the participants are in the world or not, is a social space in which people are digitally represented and so can interact, and is underpinned by networked computers that manage the world and its interactions' [3].

Many variations exist, but virtual worlds or environments are computer simulations offering some or all of the following [4]:

- Three-dimensional (3D) spaces
- People represented by avatars
- Objects in the world are persistent and may be interacted with, e.g. moveable chairs, vehicles
- Communication is usually in real time: voice, text and gesture

Immersive clinical environments (virtual clinical worlds)

Where virtual environments are used specifically for clinical purposes, they could be termed immersive clinical environments or virtual clinical worlds. Heinrichs [3, 5] proposed that in clinical practice virtual worlds are being deployed because they offer the following beneficial attributes:

- Presence
- Immersion, i.e. engagement
- Team-based activities
- Real workplace settings
- Safe 'play spaces'
- Relatively low cost (compared to custom healthcare game development)

We now explore virtual patients, before moving on to examine how virtual patients can work within virtual worlds.

Virtual patients

'Virtual patients' (VP) is a catch-all term for a range of distinct approaches: 'Such approaches include case presentations, interactive patient scenarios, virtual patient games, human standardised patients, high fidelity software simulations, high fidelity manikins and virtual conversational agents' [6].

Kononowicz et al. [7] have adapted and refined Talbot's earlier virtual patient framework [6] to provide a more complete picture of this confusing area. He classifies VPs by competency and by technology (Table 10.1).

The focus of this chapter is on the classes 'VP games' and 'High-fidelity software simulation'. These virtual

patients are entirely computer based and should not be confused with simulated (standardized) patients; that is, humans playing the role of patients (see Chapter 7), nor with high-fidelity computer simulators connected to realistic robot mannequins [8].

Interactive virtual patients in immersive clinical environments

From Talbot [6] we recognize the components of interactive virtual patients (IVPs) as:

- A 3D clinical environment
- A human physiology engine
- 3D avatars
- Data displays
- Medical procedure capability
- Reporting or assessment capabilities

However, most of the few virtual patient models available for deployment in virtual environments are execute only; that is, they run from start to finish and cannot be interrupted or even in most cases parameterized simply at the start time. Two types of virtual patient designs can be distinguished: a *'narrative' or passive structure* and a *'problem-solving' or active structure*. In the narrative/passive cases, the simulation represents a single medical state, often in considerable detail, and with relevant graphics, audio and visual media displaying the patient's medical condition. Fewer simulations support the evolution of the 'problem-solving'/active patient state, both with and without medical intervention. In the problem-solving/active model, one specifies both gradual changes in physiological variables as well as a number of discrete important 'states', with the patient moving from state to state based on the virtual patient's condition and on the actions taken by the learner. 'Passive' patients, however, are often experienced as 'pale imitations of real world patients' [9].

The deployment of virtual environments and interactive virtual patients in healthcare is addressed in later sections.

Virtual environments and interactive virtual patients: some examples in healthcare

Healthcare is much wider than the core clinical professions. The allied healthcare professions make up 60% of the total health workforce of many millions [10] and, according to one source, 'one in every 11 attributes, as well as a taxonomy of pedagogies based on the learner/instructor dichotomy. Robbins then proposes matching pedagogy types to virtual world types. Having done this, the approach is applied to the field of information systems, before a set of guidelines is offered for the implementation of virtual worlds in other domains. The approach has been further developed and refined for the clinical context [22].

Starting from the practical perspective of introducing different virtual worlds into different courses, Delwiche [23] points out that 'All virtual environments are not created equal'. He advocates that when choosing a virtual world, the key criteria to consider are accessibility, genre and extensibility:

- *Accessibility:* Is the world easy to use and understand? If not, is the additional time investment in learning to use the world appropriate to the intended use and outcomes?
- *Genre:* Is the world theme appropriate? Some virtual worlds are fantastical, game-like environments. These are therefore unlikely to be suitable for professional healthcare education. Other worlds are dull virtual office suites for corporate meetings. Again, these may be unsuitable for certain professional uses.
- *Extensibility:* Can the world be developed to design and add new scenarios? If yes, who could add those new scenarios? In other words, what level of skill and access are needed? Can the student or instructor modify the world or does it require a sophisticated C++ programmer?

In the context of professional environments in healthcare, a further factor should be added:

- *Security:* Can the virtual world be made private? Notice that this is an option, but the fact that non-public professional conversations and activities may be observed in a public virtual world is not acceptable to many healthcare organizations – and in fact to most organizations. Intruders (aka 'griefers') are never welcome!

Interactive virtual patients

Poulton [24] notes that 'Virtual Patients cannot replace real patients, but they can be of great assistance in areas where there are no other suitable learning tools, such as clinical problem solving … and arguably therefore should be an essential element of every undergraduate course'.

Virtual patients are sets of patient-linked medical data. This data can be organized into various forms:

- Linear, where the patient data is presented in a fixed, pre-determined sequence (e.g. CASUS) [25].
- Branching, where the data is structured into various paths with the student decisions on treatment affecting the patient's outcomes (e.g. Open Labyrinth) [26].
- Template-based systems, which allow the student to choose from ranges of possible data – interviews, lab data, physical examination – to reach a decision (e.g. CAMPUS) [27].
- Knowledge-based virtual patient applications, which are created dynamically from an algorithmic pathophysiological model (e.g. CliniSpace Dynapatients) [28].

Virtual patients now offer the opportunity to create and deliver experiences that teach critical thinking, diagnostic reasoning and even communication [29, 30] (see Figure 10.3).

Box 10.2 VPs in Nursing and Paramedicine

VPs were introduced as an assessment tool in three different nursing courses at two universities, comprising 77 students in total. Students' overall acceptance of this assessment tool, including its applicability to the practice of nursing and the potential of VP-based assessment as a learning experience, were investigated using questionnaires. Course directors used the Web-SP system to assess students' interactions with VPs and their answers regarding diagnoses, caring procedures and their justifications. Students found the VP cases to be realistic and engaging, and indicated a high level of acceptance for this assessment method. In addition, the students indicated that VPs were good for practising their clinical skills, although some would prefer the VP system to be less 'medical' and asked for more focus on nursing. Although most students supplied correct diagnoses and made adequate clinical decisions, there was a wide range in their ability to explain their clinical reasoning processes [32].

In a different context with paramedicine students and using the Second Life VE with the MedBiquitous VP international standard, Conradi et al. [33] reported that students believed that VEs provided a more realistic learning experience than problem-based classroom learning.

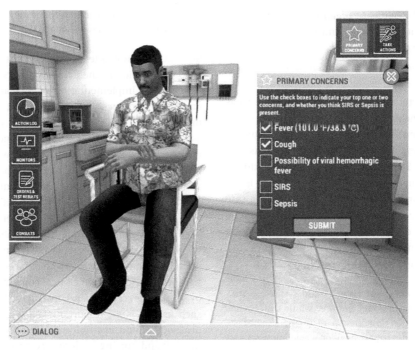

PRIMARY CONCERNS

Use the check boxes to indicate your top one or two concerns, and whether you think SIRS or Sepsis is present.

☑ Fever (101.0 °F/38.3 °C)

☑ Cough

☐ Possibility of viral hemorrhagic fever

☐ SIRS

☐ Sepsis

SUBMIT

DIALOG

Figure 10.3 Example of a virtual patient in a virtual clinical environment. Source: SimTabs [31].

Box 10.3 Comparing Mannequin-Based Simulation with Virtual Patient Simulation

A randomized controlled study with 57 nursing students was carried out in Singapore to compare mannequin-based simulation with virtual patient simulation prior to the nursing students' encounters with deteriorating ward patients. While the study did not demonstrate the superiority of virtual patient over mannequin-based simulation, the former was shown to be equally effective. However, when the resource implications of mannequin-based simulation – volumes of students, faculty time, scheduling – were compared with virtual patient simulation, then 'the flexibility, practicality, and scalability of the virtual patient simulation … appears to provide a more promising learning strategy over time than the mannequin-based simulation for refreshing clinical performance' [34].

Cook et al. [29] posed an important set of questions regarding the use of virtual patients: what is their role; how should they be designed and presented; how should VPs be integrated with other educational activities; how can they be used in assessment; and who will develop and maintain VPs?

The integration of virtual patients into realistic healthcare virtual environments is novel and, while it is now being implemented in day-to-day clinical educational situations, it is still a pioneering development.

Virtual environments and interactive virtual patients: rationale and issues

The implementation of new approaches in healthcare is never easy. It can be argued that the cautious approach is, in principle, the correct approach, as the patient is the end point of any new implementation. The precautionary principle requires that the introduction of innovative approaches should be evidence based. This section looks at the range of issues surrounding the introduction and implementation of virtual environments and virtual patients. At first sight these may appear daunting but, as these technologies become more 'user friendly', so enabling their rapid deployment in organizations and at a falling cost, they are beginning to move into the mainstream.

Key Term Definitions

Virtual environments: synchronous, persistent networks of people and environments, represented by avatars, facilitated by networked computers.

Virtual patients: case presentations, interactive patient scenarios, virtual patient games, human standardized patients, high-fidelity software simulations, high-fidelity mannequins and virtual conversational agents

References

1 Arciaga, P., Windokun, A., Calmes, D. *et al.* (2013) Board 501-Technology Innovations Abstract. Initial experience with the use of virtual simulation to teach students interprofessional education: the Charles R. Drew University (CDU) experience (submission# 863). *Simul Healthc*, **8** (6), 608.

2 Bell, M. (2008) Toward a definition of virtual worlds. *J Virtual Worlds Res*, **1** (1). doi: 10.4101/jvwr.v1i1.283

3 Heinrichs, L., Fellander-Tsai, L. and Davies, D. (2013) Clinical virtual worlds: the wider implications for professionals, in *Serious games and virtual worlds in education, professional development, and healthcare* (eds K. Bredl and W. Bösche), IGI Global, Hershey, PA.

4 Wikipedia. Virtual world [cited 1 September 2016]. Available at: https://en.wikipedia.org/wiki/Virtual_world

5 Heinrichs, W.L., Harter, P., Youngblood, P. *et al.* (2010) Training healthcare personnel for mass casualty incidents in a virtual emergency department. VED II. *Prehosp Disaster Med.*, **25** (5), 422–34.

6 Talbot, T.S. (2012) Sorting out the virtual patient: how to exploit artificial intelligence, game technology and sound educational practices to create engaging role-playing simulations. *IJGCMS*, **4** (3), 1–19.

7 Kononowicz, A.A., Zary, N., Edelbring, S. *et al.* (2015) Virtual patients – what are we talking about? A framework to classify the meanings of the term in healthcare education. *BMC Med Educ*, **15** (1), 11.

8 Kononowicz, A.A. and Hege, I. (2010) Virtual patients as a practical realisation of the e-learning idea in medicine, in *E-learning experiences and future* (ed. S. Soomro), InTech, Rijeka. doi: 10.5772/8803

9 Heinrichs, W.L., Dev, P. and Davies, D. (2014) The virtual sim centre: extending and augmenting in-house simulation centres. *BMJ Simul Technol Enhanced Learn*, **1** (Suppl 1), A12.

10 Wikipedia. Allied health professions [cited 1 September 2016]. Available at: https://en.wikipedia.org/wiki/Allied_health_professions

11 The Medica. Medical industry overview [cited 1 September 2016]. Available at: http://www.themedica.com/industry-overview.html

12 Siddiqi, S., Mama, S.K. and Lee, R.E. (2010) Developing an obesity prevention intervention in virtual worlds: the international health challenge in Second Life. *J Virtual Worlds Res*, **3** (3). doi: 10.4101/jvwr.v3i3.809

13 Ghanbarzadeh, R., Ghapanchi, A.H., Blumenstein, M. and Talaei-Khoei, A. (2014) A decade of research on the use of three-dimensional virtual worlds in health care: a systematic literature review. *J Med Internet Res*, **16** (2), e47. doi: 10.2196/jmir.3097

14 Stokowski LA. A digital revolution: games, simulations, and virtual worlds in nursing education. Medscape. 2013;15 March [cited January 2014]. Available at: http://www.medscape.com/viewarticle/780819.

15 Foronda, C., Godsall, L. and Trybulski, J. (2013) Virtual clinical simulation: the state of the science. *Clin Simul Nurs*, **9** (8), e279–e286.

16 Stewart, S. and Davis, D. (2012) On the MUVE or in decline: reflecting on the sustainability of the Virtual Birth Centre developed in Second Life. *Aust J Educ Technol*, **28** (3), 480–503.

17 Hack CJ. The benefits and barriers of using virtual worlds to engage healthcare professionals on distance learning programmes. *Interact Learn Environ*. Online before print. 2015;1–14. doi: 10.1080/10494820.2015.1057743

18 Brown, R., Rasmussen, R., Baldwin, I. and Wyeth, P. (2012) Design and implementation of a virtual world training simulation of ICU first hour handover processes. *Aust Crit Care*, **25** (3), 178–87. doi: 10.1016/j.aucc.2012.02.005

19 Flin, R. and Maran, N. (2004) Identifying and training non-technical skills for teams in acute medicine. *Qual Saf Health Care*, **13** (suppl 1), i80–i88.

20 Kim, S.H., Lee, J.L. and Thomas, M.K. (2012) Between purpose and method: a review of educational research on 3D virtual worlds. *J Virtual Worlds Res*, **5** (1).

21 Robbins, R.W. (2009) Selecting a virtual world platform for learning. *J Inform Syst Educ*, **20** (2), 199–210.

22 Davies, D., Arciaga, P., Dev, P. and Heinrichs, W.L. (2015) Interactive virtual patients in immersive clinical environments: the potential for learning, in *Simulations in medicine* (ed. I. Roterman-Konieczna), Walter De Gruyter, Berlin, pp. 138–78.

23 Delwiche, A. (2006) Massively multiplayer online games (MMOs) in the new media classroom. *J Educ Technol Soc*, **9** (3), 160–72.

24 Poulton, T. (2011) Virtual patients: a year of change. *Med Teach*, **33** (11), 933–7.

25 Fischer, M.R. (2000) CASUS: An authoring and learning tool supporting diagnostic reasoning, in *Use of computers in medical education (part II)*. *Zeitschrift für Hochschuldidaktik*, vol. **1** (ed. C. Daetwyler), pp. 87–98.

26 SourceForge. Open Labyrinth [cited 30 July 2015]. Available at: http://sourceforge.net/projects/openlabyrinth

27 Garde, S., Heid, J., Haag, M. *et al.* (2007) Can design principles of traditional learning theories be fulfilled by computer-based training systems in medicine: the example of CAMPUS. *Int J Med Inform*, **76** (2–3), 124–9.

28 Heinrichs, L., Dev, P. and Davies, D. (2015) (2015) Authoring, deploying, and managing dynamic virtual patients in virtual clinical environments. *BAMS*, **11** (2), 79–88.

29 Cook, D.A., Erwin, P.J. and Triola, M.M. (2010) Computerized virtual patients in health professions education: a systematic review and meta-analysis. *Acad Med*, **85** (10), 1589–602.

30 Dev, P. (2015) Simulation: a view into the future of education, in *Healthcare information management systems: cases, strategies, and solutions*, 4th edn (eds M.J. Ball, C.A. Weaver, G.R. Kim and J.M. Kiel), Springer, Berlin, pp. 317–29.

31 Simtabs. [cited 1 September 2016]. Available at: http://simtabs.com/

32 Forsberg, E., Georg, C., Ziegert, K. and Fors, U. (2011) Virtual patients for assessment of clinical reasoning in nursing: a pilot study. *Nurs Educ Today*, **31** (8), 757–62.

33 Conradi, E., Kavia, S., Burden, D. *et al.* (2009) Virtual patients in a virtual world: training paramedic students for practice. *Med Teach*, **31** (8), 713–20.

34 Liaw, S.Y., Chan, S.W.C., Chen, F.G. *et al.* (2014) Comparison of virtual patient simulation with mannequin-based simulation for improving clinical performances in assessing and managing clinical deterioration: randomized controlled trial. *J Med Internet Res*, **16** (9).

35 Cooke, M., Irby, D.M., Sullivan, W. and Ludmerer, K.M. (2006) American medical education 100 years after the Flexner report. *N Engl J Med*, **355** (13), 1339–44.

36 Hayden, J.K., Smiley, R.A., Alexander, M. *et al.* (2014) The NCSBN National Simulation Study: a longitudinal, randomized, controlled study replacing clinical hours with simulation in prelicensure nursing education. *J Nurs Reg*, **5** (2 Suppl), S3–S64.

37 Gregory, S., Scutter, S., Jacka, L. *et al.* (2015) Barriers and enablers to the use of virtual worlds in higher education: an exploration of educator perceptions, attitudes and experiences. *J Educ Technol Soc*, **18** (1), 3–12.

38 Heinrichs, W.L. (2008) Simulation for team training and assessment: case studies of online training with virtual worlds. *World J Surg.*, **2**, 161–70.

39 Heinrichs, W.L., Davies, D. and Davies, J. (2012) Virtual worlds in healthcare: applications and implications, in *Serious games for healthcare: applications and implications* (eds S. Arnab, I. Dunwell and K. Debattista), IGI Global, Hershey, PA, pp. 1–22.

40 McDonald, M., Gregory, S., Farley, H. *et al.* (2014) Coming of the third wave: a move toward best practice, user defined tools and mainstream integration for virtual worlds in education, in *Proceedings of the 31st Australasian Society for Computers in Learning in Tertiary Education Conference (ASCILITE 2014). (pp. 161-170)*, Macquarie University, Sydney, pp. 161–70.

41 CliniSpace. Virtual Sim Center [cited 1 September 2016]. Available at: http://virtualsimcenter.clinispace.com/

42 Wikipedia. Oculus Rift [cited 1 September 2016]. Available at: https://en.wikipedia.org/wiki/Oculus_Rift

43 Wikipedia. Windows Holographic [cited 1 September 2016]. Available at: https://en.wikipedia.org/wiki/Windows_Holographic#Microsoft_HoloLens

CHAPTER 11

Consistency in simulation: A measurement perspective

Brian Jolly

KEY MESSAGES

- There are 3 different measurement strategies that can be of assistance in developing and running simulations.

- The first, event validity, is simply the explicit comparison, over a series of iterations of the simulation, of the events resulting from the simulation to those that occurred in the real-life situation on which the simulation is based.

- The second, Generalizability Theory, should become one of the standard analytical techniques for studies of the impact of simulation and its use as an assessment tool.

- The third, Rasch scaling, could be used to classify the difficulty of simulations on a scale, or to build a taxonomy of simulations.

- Although many simulations are imperfect, they nevertheless are useful tools with established validity evidence that may, in a relatively short time, augment or replace workplace-based learning.

Overview

The use of simulation in healthcare education has been expanding since the early 1970s. Recently the pace of development has increased rapidly, as the result of technological advances and significant investment from government and business sectors. Narratives of these many developments are included in this book. Although there has been much interest in the measurement of elements of the simulation environment, and the replication of specific experiences or simulated parameters through computer control and other means, relatively little attention has been paid to what metrics can be used to capture the value, difficulty and performance of the

elements of the simulations we use. This chapter makes some suggestions, from among many alternatives, around how recent developments in psychometrics can be used to measure simulation characteristics. What we still lack is a complete taxonomy of simulation, and this book may contribute to its development.

Introduction

Using simulation is a valuable strategy to create learning activities and events that cannot usually be guaranteed to take place in the course of day-to-day clinical placements. Simulation can be used as a means of ensuring that health professionals have basic skills, such as taking blood, examining ears or soft tissue therapy, that can be learnt without subjecting patients to excessive risk from novice practitioners. It has also been used extensively in the development of assessments at both undergraduate and advanced levels in a wide range of professions, including medicine, nursing and police training [1–3]. In the early days of simulated patient (SP) development, a large number of papers were written about the effectiveness of the methodology, employed as both a teaching and an assessment strategy, without authors paying very much attention to reporting the characteristics and development of the simulation itself [4]. For example, details about the repeatability of SP performance, and the style and length of the training involved, were often absent entirely from some reports of projects involving SPs [4]. Furthermore, because SPs were generally very much like real patients, the validity of the experience from the learner's perspective was often assumed, rather than critically examined.

Healthcare Simulation Education: Evidence, Theory and Practice, First Edition.
Edited by Debra Nestel, Michelle Kelly, Brian Jolly and Marcus Watson.
© 2018 John Wiley & Sons Ltd. Published 2018 by John Wiley & Sons Ltd.

Particularly in the assessment mode, the issue of measurement has been prominent, but often the assessment instruments used in these simulations have taken a back seat to the focus on the simulation activity. In this chapter we will outline three different measurement strategies that can be of assistance in developing and running simulations, and in using data from those simulations in an assessment and/or developmental capacity.

Simulation event validity

In a classic early paper on the validity of simulation, Hermann [5] identified this lack of testing the assumptions in the following terms:

> Probably no approach to model validity is reported more frequently than the subjective estimates of experimenters or observers or human participants as to the correspondence between the model's operation and their perception of the actual phenomena which the game or simulation represent. (p. 221)

Hermann proposed a set of criteria for simulation validity, some of which focused on the internal structure of the simulation. This is important to recognize, as the current interest still seems to be very much in how participants perceive the simulation rather than what actually happens. One of these internal parameters Hermann termed *event validity*. Event validity is simply the comparison, over a series of iterations of the simulation, of the events resulting from the simulation to those that occurred in the real-life situation on which the simulation is based. This is primarily a qualitative endeavour; the details of the originating event are written down, and each time the simulation is used, the events unfolding are also recorded. Over time these data will give rise to a frequency distribution of events, some of which may be the intended outcomes and some of which may be quite novel and/or disruptive. If these novel or disruptive events are too frequent, the simulation may be suffering from some corruptive influences. When Hermann wrote his original paper, the availability of computing power was such that these recordings would have been a tedious and cumbersome process. With today's sophisticated programming and laptop/tablet capabilities, augmented by voice-to-text

conversion software, there is the possibility of generating these comparisons and databases quite easily. Although validation of simulations is extensively used in computer models of real events [6], and many of the methods used are not applicable to healthcare educational simulations, event validity is one of those that has utility.

The importance of event validity to the use of simulation in assessment tasks should not be underestimated. Subtle changes in the simulation arising from any number of sources could result in different outcomes in the simulation. Candidate behaviours related to the intended outcomes may be inhibited by such changes, and replaced by behaviours that do not attract a value or a score within the simulation. Given that someone who may not have been involved with the station's generation, or the training that the SP received, often scores simulations within the objective structured clinical examinations (OSCEs) as a kind of fly-in, fly-out assessor, this increases the likelihood that these changes will go unnoticed. Recording data for the event validity comparison can reduce this effect. It is also useful from time to time to benchmark performance in the simulation by getting an expert to undertake the simulation, just to confirm that, in such circumstances, the appropriate events do take place.

Other approaches to reliability in simulation

Two longstanding issues in the study of simulation were the difficulty of obtaining unbiased ratings of participants' performance in the simulation and the lack of an appropriate framework in which reliability or consistency could be investigated. The event validity already described goes some way to overcoming the issue of consistency across different iterations of a simulation event, as far as outcomes are concerned. However, there are still issues of measurement consistency when SPs contribute ratings to the assessment process, as well as biases transmitted by the perspectives of assessors (whether SPs or faculty) and the complex issue of *case specificity*. Case specificity is the persistent phenomenon that the performance of students and trainees varies substantially from case to case, even though the same so-called generic skills (e.g. history taking) are used across all cases [7]. In a simulated scenario, there is the added unpredictability that not only do the cases differ, the precise way in which they are portrayed by different SPs may also differ, and the variance introduced by the SP (as both actor and assessor in some cases) may enlarge or reduce the variability across cases. This introduces another layer of complexity into the measurement situation.

Reliability or consistency of performance in the simulation

As discussed elsewhere [8], a candidate's score in an assessment based on simulation will have a number of sources of variance: the candidate themselves; the particular case; the assessor; the simulated patient; and the interaction between all these components. Where the purpose of the assessment is to rank the candidates in order of ability, ideally the candidate should be the largest source of variance. In these complex measurement situations, a common procedure is to look at the intercorrelation of the measures. For example, several observers or instruments may be used to assess the events in a simulation, or a suite of simulations, on different occasions, involving several different SPs and so on. All the different measures would be intercorrelated with each other, producing a large matrix of correlation coefficients. However, this is a very inefficient way of using these data.

Those methods have been supplanted in recent years by a technique called generalizability or G theory [9, 10]. In this technique we make use of all the data to quantify all sources of error (candidate, case, assessor, SP and interactions between these components) and their relative contribution to the candidates' variance in scores. Then the actual values of these variances (called variance components) for each variable are combined to express the extent to which differences between candidates reflect reproducible differences. This results in a coefficient between 0 and 1, called the generalizability coefficient (G). A value for G of 0.8 is the accepted level of reliability required for a high-stakes assessment. In addition, the data can be used to model what the most efficient assessment strategy would be. For example, if it were found that the variance component for SPs had a major influence on candidates' scores, this would indicate either that more training and standardization would be required for the SPs, or that a greater number of SPs (and by implication a greater number of simulations) would

be needed to assess the candidates' performance reliably.

A series of studies using G theory on simulated patients in a large-scale examination was performed in the early 1990s, with largely favourable results [11, 12]. However, many recent studies have been undertaken without using G theory. In one example [13], the authors concluded:

> Verbal portrayal by SPs did not significantly differ for most items; however, the facial expressions of the SPs differed significantly ($p < .05$). An emergency management station that depended heavily on SPs physical presentation and facial expressions differed between all four SPs trained for that station.

Yet without measuring the impact of these differences on the overall scores of candidates across the OSCE using G theory, the relative size and potential impact of the SP differences would not be accurately assessable. G theory should become one of the standard analytical techniques for studies of the impact of simulation and its use as an assessment tool. For more information on the power of generalizability analyses, see articles by Downing and Smit [14, 15].

Scaling simulations

In occupational therapy and physiotherapy, patients are frequently given tasks or exercises to do that start simple and get progressively more complex and/or intricate; a so-called hierarchy of skills. The therapeutic principle behind this is simple: patients who have had strokes or trauma injuries need to learn to do the simpler things first, and be successful at those, before going on to harder ones.

The means by which the patient tasks are organized in occupational therapy and physiotherapy is called scaling, and it is a spin-off from a branch of psychometric theory called latent trait theory [16], developed by Georg Rasch, a Danish mathematician. In latent trait theory, the ability of test takers (the stroke patient, for example) and the difficulty of the tasks are viewed as points on the same continuous latent variable or 'trait'. For example, in occupational therapy tests, 'task' parameters characterize the difficulty of tasks, while 'person' parameters exemplify the ability or attainment level of the patients who are being assessed. The higher a person's ability, relative to the difficulty of a task, the higher the probability of successful completion of that task. In Rasch terms, when a patient's location on the latent trait is equal to the difficulty of the task, there is, by definition, a 50% chance of a successful response. When applied to tasks of varying complexity, this simple principle allows the tasks to be arranged along a continuous scale.

In the health sciences, patient-reported outcomes are often used for assessment of clinical trials, where measures of patient improvement and/or deterioration are required. Rasch analysis underpins this concept, providing a transformation of an ordinal score into a linear, interval-level variable. Originally developed for use with dichotomous items (i.e. right/wrong), it has been applied to items with a greater bandwidth. In addition, it has been applied to constellations of items that are much more complex and relate to ratings that might be seen as multidimensional. (The original idea was that the items should link together in a unidimensional fashion. However, enough work has been done with multifaceted items to suggest that the technique is applicable, as long as the items are also 'held together' in particular constellations by an umbrella concept such as maturation, rehabilitation recovery from stroke, or remission from psychiatric illness.)

The Rasch measurement model is now established as the psychometric approach to outcome scales. It provides a useful tool for bringing coherence to the key issues of unidimensionality and category ordering, within the framework of measurement science. The basic strategy of the Rasch approach is to assume that the construct under study is unidimensional and then to look for evidence to disprove that assumption. It turns out that this evidence is harder to find than one would think, which makes Rasch scaling both possible and useful in a wide range of contexts.

One of the benefits claimed for simulation as a learning strategy is that it allows the degree of challenge for the student to be titrated against their ability or year level. However, the design of these simulated tasks can be quite a complex process and there is not necessarily a coherent approach to their planning and delivery.

Using Rasch analysis for simulation event monitoring or assessment scales may be very productive in being able to develop scales for particular simulations that would allow much greater control over the educational frameworks and strategies that we use in healthcare [17].

Take the example of 'non-technical' or professional skills, a recent addition to the curriculum in specialty colleges in medicine [18]. These often diverse techniques and skills include, for example, patient advocacy, graded assertiveness, empathic utterances, negotiation, situational awareness, communication, decision making and leadership/teamwork. Each could be broken down into components, and these could then be subjected to Rasch scaling using data from the simulations to address each one. These data could then be used to order those simulation events into a hierarchy that would allow participants success at basic skills before being engaged in quite complex tasks. It would also allow scaling of different combinations of modality in hybrid simulations.

Disadvantages and advantages of simulators in assessment

Some cautions have been issued about the use of simulations for presenting 'real-time' data within a scenario. This is, in a sense, a specific example of the event validity that Hermann described. Gilpin et al. [19] highlight the relative lack of data on the accuracy of the physiological models used as part of simulations of human function, suggesting that some studies reveal that these models can be inaccurate. They identified that such simulations can be based on two different modes of operation: *static models*, in which various different rhythms, such as electrocardiogram traces, are stored and then virtually cut and pasted into the simulation; and *deductive models*, in which an underlying algorithm drives the appearance of the data on the output from the mannequin, or hybrid computer/human, simulator. They point out that 'a direct consequence of using "static" datasets is that when the simulator switches from one dataset to another the transition may appear unrealistic or jerky' (p. 703). However, the algorithmic approach requires much greater insight around the real physiological functioning of patients, both from the simulation designers and from the participants in the simulation. The 'static' datasets also do not allow the simulation to reflect the changing nature of clinical conditions, where anomalous information or vacillations in the clinical picture being presented take place. Therefore, they might only assess relatively simple skills or pattern recognition, and not the capacity to respond to fluctuating patterns of data.

Nevertheless, Gilpin et al. [19] do point to a situation in the not too distant future where computer algorithmic and data-based physiological simulations will be highly tuned to real events, and will need to be delivered by clinicians with the expert knowledge to manage a simulation that is as subtle and complex as real life.

In other domains evidence is rapidly emerging that simulation-based assessments often correlate positively with patient-related outcomes. Recent meta-analyses by Dawe et al. and Brydges et al. [20, 21], only two of a number emerging in recent years, suggest that although many simulations are imperfect, they nevertheless are useful tools with established validity evidence that may, in a relatively short time, replace workplace-based learning and assessment for select procedural skills, and maybe much more.

Key term definitions

Event validity: A parameter of simulation that indicates the frequency with which events within the real-life scenario on which the simulation is based occur within the simulated event. These frequencies are sometimes compared with the frequencies of extraneous events within the simulation.

Generalizability theory: A statistical framework for conceptualizing, investigating and designing reliable observations. It is used to determine the reliability (i.e. reproducibility) of measurements under specific conditions.

Rasch analysis: A unique approach of mathematical modelling based on a latent trait that accomplishes measurement of persons and items on the same scale, so that item values are calibrated and person abilities are measured on a shared continuum that accounts for the latent trait. In simulation terms the latent trait might be the ability to place a catheter in a simulated vein, or the ability to manage a rapid response team.

Scaling: The capacity to place a series of items, tests or tasks on a continuous scale, for example of difficulty, complexity or value.

Simulated patient: A well person role playing a patient, for the purposes of learning and/or assessment.

References

1 Pugh, D., Hamstra, S.J., Wood, T.J. *et al.* (2015) A procedural skills OSCE: assessing technical and non-technical skills of internal medicine residents. *Adv Health Sci Educ*, **20** (1), 85–100.

2 Mitchell, M.L., Henderson, A., Jeffrey, C. *et al.* (2015) Application of best practice guidelines for OSCEs: an Australian evaluation of their feasibility and value. *Nurs Educ Today*, **35** (5), 700–5.

3 Blair I, Broughton F, Burden T et al. *Police Leadership Development Board Appendix*. London: Policing and Reducing Crime Unit; 2001. Available at: http://policeauthority.org/Metropolitan/downloads/committees/previous/x-hr/hr-010621-12-appendices.pdf

4 Jolly, B. (1982) A review of issues in live patient simulation. *Innov Educ Train Int*, **19** (2), 99–107.

5 Hermann, C.F. (1967) Validation problems in games and simulations with special reference to models of international politics. *Behav Sci.*, **12**, 216–31.

6 Sargent, R.G. (2013) Verification and validation of simulation models. *J Simul.*, **7**, 12–24.

7 Wimmers, P.F. and Fung, C.C. (2008) The impact of case specificity and generalisable skills on clinical performance: a correlated traits–correlated methods approach. *Med Educ*, **42** (6), 580–8.

8 Weller, J.M., Robinson, B.J., Jolly, B. *et al.* (2005) Psychometric characteristics of simulation-based assessment in anaesthesia and accuracy of self-assessed scores. *Anaesthesia*, **60** (3), 245–50.

9 Weller, J.M., Jolly, B. and Robinson, B. (2008) Generalisability of behavioural skills in simulated anaesthetic emergencies. *Anaesthes Intensive Care*, **36** (2), 185.

10 Crossley, J., Humphris, G. and Jolly, B. (2002) Assessing health professionals. *Med Educ*, **36** (9), 800–4.

11 Tamblyn, R.M., Klass, D.J., Schnabl, G.R. and Kopelow, M.L. (1991) The accuracy of standardized patient presentation. *Med Educ.*, **25**, 100–9.

12 Tamblyn, R., Klass, D.J., Schnabl, G.R. and Kopelow, M.L. (1991) Sources of unreliability and bias in standardized patient ratings. *Teach Learn Med.*, **3**, 74–85.

13 Baig, L.A., Beran, T.N., Vallevand, A. *et al.* (2014) Accuracy of portrayal by standardized patients: results from four OSCE stations conducted for high stakes examinations. *BMC Med Educ.*, **14**, 97. doi: 10.1186/1472-6920-14-97

14 Downing, S.M. (2004) Reliability: on the reproducibility of assessment data. *Med Educ*, **38** (9), 1006–12.

15 Smit, G.N. and Van Der Molen, H.T. (1997) The construction and evaluation of simulations to assess professional interviewing skills. *Assess Educ*, **4** (3), 353–64.

16 Tennant, A. and Conaghan, P.G. (2007) The Rasch measurement model in rheumatology: what is it and why use it? When should it be applied, and what should one look for in a Rasch paper? *Arthr Rheum.*, **57**, 1358–62. doi: 10.1002/art.23108

17 Hancock, N., Bundy, A., Honey, A. *et al.* (2011) Improving measurement properties of the Recovery Assessment Scale with Rasch analysis. *Am J Occup Ther*, **65** (6), e77–e85.

18 Royal Australasian College of Surgeons. Non-technical skills for surgeons (NOTSS) [cited 1 September 2016]. Available at: http://www.surgeons.org/for-health-professionals/register-courses-events/professional-development/non-technical-skills-for-surgeons/

19 Gilpin, K., Pybus, D.A. and Vuylsteke, A. (2012) Medical simulation in 'my world'. *Anaesthesia.*, **67**, 702–5.

20 Dawe, S.R., Pena, G.N., Windsor, J.A. *et al.* (2014) Systematic review of skills transfer after surgical simulation-based training. *Br J Surg.*, **101**, 1063–76.

21 Brydges, R., Hatala, R., Zendejas, B. *et al.* (2015) Linking simulation-based educational assessments and patient-related outcomes: a systematic review and meta-analysis. *Acad Med*, **90** (2), 246–56.

CHAPTER 12

Taking simulation beyond education in healthcare

Marcus Watson

Overview

This chapter explores the broader roles of healthcare simulation. It discusses the use of simulation in other industries that require first aid and emergency response skills. It expands on the application of simulation in healthcare to include recruitment, career development and patient advocacy. The chapter also looks into the emerging use of simulation as a therapeutic intervention.

Healthcare education using simulation for non-healthcare industries

As the capacity for healthcare simulation grows with the increasing number of facilities, advances in evidence and technologies, so too do those areas in which simulation can be applied. This chapter aims to be thought provoking as to the future uses for simulation in those settings.

The most elementary extension of healthcare simulation is its application to education and training outside of traditional healthcare contexts. Many industries require some level of first aid training; however, some industries require more advanced medical emergency response skills. Industries including defence, mining, manufacturing, aviation and maritime often outsource training and this provides opportunities for simulation facilities. In many cases the industries have accredited training where simulation could be integrated to meet some or all of the requirements of a programme. In other cases specialized training is sought to meet an emerging need. For example, the outbreak of Ebola had a range of industries scrambling for training on the use of personal protective equipment. Another opportunity for various industries is to use medical emergency response training as a team-building exercise. Equally there are opportunities to work with and inform other industries in skills such as simulation facilitation and scenario design.

Many healthcare simulation facilities experience fluctuations in demand for their services from hospitals and tertiary education institutes. With appropriate scheduling, the training of non-healthcare industries has the potential to bring in significant funding that can then be applied to the healthcare simulation facilities' core business. Such training also provides opportunities to get external assessment of a simulation process, including training, assessment and management. It is also possible for the training of people from other industries to increase the opportunity to conduct research on the efficacy of simulation, since many people may be

Healthcare Simulation Education: Evidence, Theory and Practice, First Edition.
Edited by Debra Nestel, Michelle Kelly, Brian Jolly and Marcus Watson.
© 2018 John Wiley & Sons Ltd. Published 2018 by John Wiley & Sons Ltd.

novices with no prior experience that could influence learning outcomes.

Knowledge and skills development beyond the clinical context: life skills

Simulation in healthcare has a focus on clinical skills for individuals and teams. In some cases simulation facilities have been used to expand beyond clinical skills to help people choose careers and develop non-clinical skills required in the effective running of hospitals and health services. Gaba describes simulation being used from 'cradle to grave', including with school children and members of the lay public, to explain healthcare issues and practices, educate people in basic sciences and engage the interest of students in clinical careers [1].

Using simulation to recruit future healthcare professionals

It is predicted, with the world's population ageing, that healthcare and social assistance are going to be the largest areas of employment growth [2]. Choosing a career in the modern world is difficult for young people, given that many jobs of the future have not yet been created. Furthermore, subject choice in mid-secondary schooling may have an impact on tertiary entry opportunities, especially in healthcare. In many industries, work experience can provide school students with some insight into what a career might offer. Traditional work experience in healthcare is exceptionally limited, as it would be inappropriate for children to undertake the activities conducted by doctors, nurses or other healthcare professionals. Well-designed simulations can act as an alternative to work experience, where young students can get hands-on experience that would normally only occur some time into a professional career. They also provide the ability for students to experience several professions in a short amount of time.

Using simulation to advocate healthcare

Simulation can provide powerful narratives (Chapter 8) and compelling experiences (Chapter 4) that can be used to motivate people to change their behaviour. Simulation has been used in many campaigns to address the causes of trauma, such as drink driving; however, more recently simulation has been used to address behaviours with long-term consequences, such as the

APRIL® Face Aging Software, which simulates the effect of smoking on ageing [3]. Alternatively, using make-up 'moulage' showing the impact of smoking on age has also been employed [4]. Simulation also has the ability to help carers and clinicians experience illness from the patient's perspective. The Virtual Dementia Experience™ has won awards for the use of game technology to deliver experiential learning [5]. As virtual and augmented reality technologies advance over the next five to ten years, the breadth of applications for health advocacy is likely to expand rapidly.

Using simulation for leadership development

In team-based clinical training, the leadership role is often a core component of scenarios and debriefing. Programs such as Crisis Resource Management focus on leadership, role clarity and good teamwork; however, broader leadership skills are likely to be required to undertake other roles in healthcare successfully. For example, the skills required to lead a sustainable department over years will go beyond those faced in most traditional clinical scenarios. Again, the use of persuasive experiences (Chapter 4) and strong narratives (Chapter 8) can create financial, human resources and ethical scenarios to develop future healthcare leaders.

Applying simulation to design and evaluation in healthcare

Healthcare is getting more complex, with the average lag in translational research estimated at 17 years [6]. The general consensus is that we need to get new technologies and therapies into healthcare quicker than we have historically. Simulation has the potential to play a role between bench top and bedside, in analysing both what works and also how best to implement changes in practice. Further simulations can be used to understand and improve the way we deliver care and even how we design facilities and processes of care.

Using simulation as a diagnostic tool (immersive and modelling)

Simulation can be used to examine existing processes and technologies to identify better ways to deliver care. Simulation has already been used to evaluate new technologies prior to clinical trials. These vary from new ways of representing information for graphical cardiovascular display [6, 7] through to new devices for displaying information [8]. Equally, simulation has been used to understand and improve the delivery of clinical processes. Employing discrete event simulation as a prototype, the simulation showed that a minor rotation among the nurses could reduce the mean number of visitors that had to be referred to alternative flows within the hospital from 87 to 37 on a daily basis, well within the work capacity of the staff [9]. Another study that placed simulated patients in a real clinical setting reduced the mean time for chest pain (STEMI) patients to arrive at the cardiovascular lab for treatment by 55% [10]. Both modelling simulation and immersive simulation have proven effective for improving existing processes of care. More examples are discussed in Chapter 5.

Using simulation as a predictive tool

Both computer-based models and immersive simulations also have a role to play as predictive tools for healthcare. One area that is expanding is the use of computer simulations to model pharmacology for decision support systems in order to guide clinical decision making [11]. Such decision support systems are likely to change the way clinicians practise and therefore to have an impact on the technologies and processes used in simulation. Chapter 5 provides a more detailed discussion of where predictive simulation can be used to understand how new technologies might change the way clinicians need to practise.

Simulation as therapy

The ability to design simulations that engage through narrative, meaning and entertainment means that simulation may work where traditional approaches fail. Simulations using virtual environments are now demonstrating effectiveness for cognitive and motor skill rehabilitation. Areas such as fear reduction [12], therapy for combat-related post-traumatic stress disorder [13], pain reduction during wound care and physical therapy with burn patients [14] have demonstrated the value of virtual reality simulation for patient care. It has also been argued that video games can be used to improve adherence to physiotherapy programmes [15]. Simulation as a therapy may not work for all patients,

however; for example, some patients might find the technology threatening and therefore fail to engage with the simulation.

As the virtual environments improve, so do the interfaces, including motion sensing input devices (e.g. Kinect) and voice recognition, which will expand the types of solutions that can be created. With the bourgeoning accessibility to virtual reality and the introduction of augmented reality, it is likely that simulation will become one of many tools clinicians have at their disposal to meet patient needs. It is tempting to think (as it is with all forms of simulation) that higher levels of realism will provide better outcomes. Potentially well-designed, simple simulations (both virtual and physical) will achieve as much or more than expensive virtual environments. The development of therapeutic simulations will require significant research to ensure that they go beyond engagement and produce improved patient outcomes. As much of that research will need to be developed, how do we use simulation to train clinicians to apply therapeutic simulations effectively?

Conclusion

This chapter has aired some alternative uses of simulation beyond traditional clinical education and training. As technology and evidence build in healthcare, the use of simulation will diversify, which will broaden both opportunities and challenges for simulation providers. As many of the reports of using simulation beyond education in healthcare exist in the grey literature, there is a need to formalize research and share learning across healthcare.

References

1 Gaba, D.M. (2004) The future vision of simulation in health care. *Qual Saf Health Care.*, **13**, i2–i10. doi: 10.1136/qshc.2004.009878
2 Australian Workforce and Productivity Agency. *Future focus: 2013 National Workforce Development Strategy.* Canberra: Commonwealth of Australia; 2013. Available at: https://docs.education.gov.au/system/files/doc/other/futurefocus2013nwds-2013.pdf
3 Burford, O., Moyez Jiwa, B., Carter, O. *et al.* (2013) Internet-based photoaging within Australian pharmacies to promote smoking cessation: randomized controlled trial. *J Med Internet Res*, **15** (3), e64.

4 Queensland Government. See the ugly side of smoking [cited 1 September 2016]. Available at: http://ifyousmoke.initiatives.qld.gov.au/

5 Alzheimer's Australia. Virtual Dementia Experience [cited 1 September 2016]. Available at: https://vic.fightdementia.org.au/vic/about-us/virtual-dementia-experience

6 Albert, R.W., Agutter, J.A., Syroid, N.D. *et al.* (2007) A simulation-based evaluation of a graphic cardiovascular display. *Anesth Analg*, **105** (5), 1303–11.

7 Sanderson, P.M., Watson, M.O., Russell, W.J. *et al.* (2008) Advanced auditory displays and head mounted displays: advantages and disadvantages for monitoring by the distracted anesthesiologist. *Anesthes Analges*, **106** (6), 1787–97.

8 David, L., Jenkins, S.A., Sanderson, P.M. *et al.* (2010) Monitoring with head-mounted displays in general anesthesia: a clinical evaluation in the operating room. *Anaesthes Analges*, **110** (4), 1032–8.

9 Nielsen, A.L., Hilwig, H., Kissoon, N. and Teelucksingh, S. (2008) Discrete event simulation as a tool in optimization of a professional complex adaptive system. *Stud Health Technol Inform.*, **136**, 247–52.

10 Cullen, L., Brazil, V., Dooris, M., Baldwin, M. and Muller, H. (2012). 'Stemi-sim'—A 'Process of Care' simulation can help improve door to balloon times for patients with ST elevation myocardial infarction. *Heart, Lung and Circulation*, **21**, p.S50.

11 Barrett, J.S., Mondick, J.T., Narayan, M. *et al.* (2008) Integration of modeling and simulation into hospital-based decision support systems guiding pediatric pharmacotherapy. *BMC Med Inform Decis Mak.*, **8**, 6. doi: 10.1186/1472-6947-8-6

12 Parsons, T.D. and Rizzo, A.A. (2008) Affective outcomes of virtual reality exposure therapy for anxiety and specific phobias: a meta-analysis. *J Behav Ther Exper Psychiatry.*, **39**, 250–61.

13 Rothbaum, B.O., Rizzo, A.S. and Difede, J. (2010) Virtual reality exposure therapy for combat-related posttraumatic stress disorder. *Ann N Y Acad Sci.*, **1208**, 126–32. doi: 10.1111/j.1749-6632.2010.05691.x

14 Hoffman, H.G., Chambers, G.T., Meyer, W.J. *et al.* (2011) Virtual reality as an adjunctive non-pharmacologic analgesic for acute burn pain during medical procedures. *Ann Behav Med*, **41** (2), 183–91.

15 Lohse, K., Shirzad, N., Verster, A. *et al.* (2013) Video games and rehabilitation: using design principles to enhance engagement in physical therapy. *J Neurol Phys Ther*, **37** (4), 166–75. doi: 10.1097/NPT.0000000000000017

CHAPTER 13

The value of professional societies to the healthcare simulation community of practice

Pamela B. Andreatta, Kirsty J. Freeman & Ralph J. MacKinnon

KEY MESSAGES

- How discipline-specific organizations support healthcare simulation interest groups within their broader mission has impacts on the development of simulation.

- Professional associations whose primary membership comprises healthcare simulation specialists from one professional discipline or another are developing rapidly.

- Professional associations whose primary membership comprises healthcare simulation specialists from multiple professional disciplines tend to operate at national and international levels.

- It helps to understand the development and role of simulation organizations if we use some theoretical perspectives on them derived from the field of educational anthropology, using the concept of 'communities of practice'.

- There are three key elements that are integral to all communities of practice: the domain, the practice and the community.

- Discipline-specific professional societies provide the opportunity for individuals to network and collaborate with others who have common interests in a shared domain expertise.

- Within these, special interest groups on simulation support the social aspects of professional identity and provide a common contextual framework for those using simulation in a particular domain, and the opportunity to engage others' awareness of simulation methodologies.

- Single-discipline simulation societies add tremendous value by developing techniques, libraries of shared resources and best-practice guidelines for the implementation of simulation in their professional discipline.

- The disadvantages of discipline-specific groups are the potential for a restricted viewpoint on healthcare simulation, a prescribed approach to applications and uses of simulation within the discipline, and a naivety about alternative possibilities derived from the broader simulation community.

- Multidisciplinary simulation societies provide a channel for determining which elements of discipline-specific simulation-based practices are broadly transferable on a global scale.

- The greatest benefit to the membership of all types of healthcare simulation professional societies is a strong collaborative mindset to advance the science and implementation of healthcare simulation.

Overview

This chapter describes how healthcare simulation professional societies and organizations have contributed to the development of simulation education and clinical practice over the last 20 years. It tracks the added value of single-, multi- and interdisciplinary or professional communities to this development, and analyses the strengths and limitations of each group. It summarizes the role of 18 such organizations. This narrative emphasizes the value of collaboration and synergy between educators and the health and simulation industries. Through the lens of Lave and Wenger's concept of 'communities of practice', we identify how best to deal with the limitations, and enhance the strengths, of simulation education support groups.

Healthcare Simulation Education: Evidence, Theory and Practice, First Edition.
Edited by Debra Nestel, Michelle Kelly, Brian Jolly and Marcus Watson.
© 2018 John Wiley & Sons Ltd. Published 2018 by John Wiley & Sons Ltd.

Introduction to professional societies

Professional societies are organizations comprising individuals and groups (e.g. corporations, guilds etc.) who share common interests, work domain, specialism construct, employment context or professional objectives. They serve to facilitate engagement between their members in ways that promote the community's goals, efforts, work products and services. They also serve as a point of reference for those who are not part of the professional practice area for information about the simulation community and its interests.

A professional society can serve multiple member and community needs. For example, it may oversee the activities of a particular profession, such as those encapsulated by the Endorsed Guidelines of the Australian and New Zealand College of Anaesthetists [1]. It may represent the interests of its member through advocacy, politics, and legal and financial channels, as does the American College of Surgeons [2]. Lastly, it may represent its own self-interest to maintain a privileged and powerful position as a controlling body over admission into the profession, regulation of expected member behaviours, safeguards designed to protect public interests as they overlap with those of the professional domain, and advanced public awareness of the benefits that the community provides to the society at large [3]. Professional societies are largely considered not for profit, which means that any surplus income is typically targeted at pursuing the organization's internal objectives. These may include professional development, broadening of membership privileges, expanding the numbers of members and influence in regions throughout the world, as well as those activities associated with advocacy, oversight and public representation previously noted.

Professional societies have different membership requirements. Most require membership fees that contribute to the functional operations of the society itself (e.g. staffing, administrative costs etc.), as well as towards expenses associated with mission-centred activities. Some societies have other screening criteria for members, including education, credentials, certification, records of service and experience, an ongoing financial responsibility through philanthropy or fundraising, and an ongoing commitment to serve the society in a voluntary capacity towards achieving its mission. Professional societies rely heavily on volunteer members to lead, organize and complete their work products and services. There are numerous challenges with this expectation, but for the purposes of this chapter we will focus on the value that service to a professional society brings to the membership.

Professional representation in healthcare simulation

Unlike many discipline-specific professional associations, the healthcare simulation community comprises numerous and varied professional disciplines and work-related contexts working collaboratively in a specific contextual construct: replicating actual healthcare settings to use for the acquisition and maintenance of professional abilities apart from actual healthcare settings. These include clinicians (physicians, nurses, allied health professionals etc.); clinical educators (medicine, nursing, allied health professionals etc.); human performance professionals (human factors specialists, educational psychologists etc.); engineers (biomedical, electrical, computer etc.); computer scientists (programmers, developers, virtual reality etc.); industry (healthcare, simulation, training resources etc.); health system administrators (hospital, clinic, service payer etc.); advocacy groups (patient safety, quality improvement etc.); credentialling bodies (specialism boards, licensing authorities etc.); and students training in each of these professional areas. As healthcare simulation encompasses so many professional disciplines, the needs of the community vary accordingly.

Consider the specialism of emergency medicine (EM). The perspective of clinicians in EM is that they have a unique skill set that they use to provide first-line, often time-critical, clinical care to patients with a wide variety of illnesses, injuries and other clinical presentations. Clinicians are primarily interested in how a simulated environment will allow them to learn and practise their abilities to manage unusual situations that require accurate and timely performance on rare occasions. Likewise, simulation may be useful to them for developing processes for how to work together as a team of clinical providers, where each provider serves a different role. Clinical educators perceive that the design of instructional methods that incorporate simulated EM activities leads to the transfer of abilities from the simulated context to the actual applied EM context.

Human performance professionals will be interested in how performance within the simulated EM space is measurable and useful for providing feedback that improves performance in actual applied EM. Engineers and computer scientists focus primarily on the development of new technologies and their application for creating simulated environments, both for healthcare- and non-healthcare-related contexts. Their interest in EM may be the opportunity to use a gaming platform to address specific urgent care decision making. By design, industry must focus on producing and selling resources that are useful to its intended customers working in healthcare simulation while earning a profit. Here, the ability to produce equipment, software and instructional resources targeting EM scenarios will be the primary objective. Administrators will focus largely on the costs associated with integrating simulation-based practices into their respective contexts and the relative return on investment as it relates to quality and safety for patients in the EM department. Credentialling bodies may view simulation environments as opportunities for creating and integrating performance-based assessment criteria for licensure or other credentialling uses related to the provision of EM care.

The natural consequences of having different performance needs are that each professional discipline will necessarily view the healthcare simulation space through a different lens and from a different perspective. The challenge, then, is that the respective disciplines may have a restricted view of healthcare simulation. This is apparent in the way in which healthcare simulation is considered by professional societies and the degree to which individuals engage with simulation through their professional affiliations. Some individuals may only work with the aspect associated with their professional role; that is, a clinician may only be interested in what simulated platforms support her ability to practise her suturing skills. As a result of her relatively narrow focus within healthcare simulation, she may choose to be part of special interest groups within a professional society specific to her clinical specialism. On the other hand, an educational psychologist who specializes in developing performance abilities for physicians across multiple specialisms will have a more expansive view of healthcare simulation, because he must be able to address a broad spectrum of abilities and selectively integrate or develop the simulated platforms required to measure those abilities

accurately and consistently. A professional society that comprises multidisciplinary members solely focused on the integration of healthcare simulation would be likely to be of more value to him.

We will explore the various ways in which healthcare simulation is embraced by professional associations. First, we will consider how discipline-specific organizations support healthcare simulation interest groups within their broader membership mission. Second, we will discuss professional associations where the primary membership comprises healthcare simulation specialists from one professional discipline or another. Third, we will consider professional associations where the primary membership comprises healthcare simulation specialists from multiple professional disciplines. Each of these societies has an important role to play and the respective value to members is related to the role that simulation plays in each individual member's professional context.

Discipline-specific professional societies with special interest groups

Many professional societies are designed to serve the needs of a practice community within a specific discipline. In healthcare, this community of practice may include a variety of specialisms and sub-specialisms within the discipline (e.g. clinicians, researchers, administrators, vendors etc.). Likewise, in computer science the community may include specialists with specific areas of expertise (e.g. modelling and simulation, data management etc.). However, the central focus of discipline-specific professional societies is the discipline itself, regardless of the specific specialisms and sub-specialisms that work within its boundaries. For example, a society that serves the discipline of emergency medicine may include members from medicine, nursing, allied health professions, instrument and equipment suppliers, software engineers, transportation experts and so on. Although each specialism and sub-specialism may have a different functional relationship to the discipline, their professional interests are all nonetheless aligned with the discipline as a whole. These types of professional societies often have special interest groups to support niche areas of interest within the discipline (e.g. simulation).

The academic pediatric association (APA): simulation SIG

The vision of the Academic Pediatric Association (APA) is to create a better world for children and families by advancing child health and well-being through the work of its members and collaborators. The APA has a formalized special interest group (SIG) in simulation-based medical education, with clearly outlined mission, vision and goal statements that support those of the parent organization. The SIG is promoted as a forum in which issues related to the national simulation agenda can be disseminated and as an opportunity for APA members to network and share ideas and resources related to simulation-based practices. In this framework, the Simulation SIG focuses on how simulation relates to the defined mission of APA, rather than healthcare simulation in a broader sphere [4].

Association for medical education in europe: simulation committee

The Association for Medical Education in Europe (AMEE) is an international society that promotes excellence in healthcare education, from undergraduate to postgraduate medical education and through to continuing professional activities. AMEE aspires to support educators and their institutions in their prescribed educational activities, but also in the development of new approaches to curriculum planning, teaching and learning methods, assessment techniques and educational management. To assist in meeting its mission, AMEE formed a Simulation Committee charged with providing advice on how it could engage with and promote simulation-based teaching and assessment, including the development of resources and other materials to support the broader membership. Like the APA Simulation SIG, the objectives of the AMEE Simulation Committee serve as a subset of the larger AMEE mission [5].

Association for computing machinery (ACM): special interest group on simulation and modeling (SIM)

The Association for Computing Machinery (ACM) is the world's largest educational and scientific computing society that serves its members and the computing profession with leading-edge publications, conferences and career resources, including the computing field's premier digital library. Its mission is to deliver resources designed to advance computing as a science and a profession. The ACM SIG on Simulation and Modeling (SIM) aims to promote and disseminate the advancement of high-quality, state-of-the-art modelling and simulation (M&S) across a broad range of interests and disciplines. SIGSIM's primary objective is to develop the M&S Knowledge Repository (MSKR) as an archive and distribution channel for multimedia-delivered tutorials, educational articles, case studies, literature surveys, M&S courseware and other useful content intended for M&S professionals, analysts, managers, researchers, educators and students. In this case, the SIGSIM objectives are a direct subset of the ACM mission specifically targeting members who focus on M&S [6].

Canadian patient safety institute: canadian network for simulation in healthcare

The mission of the Canadian Patient Safety Institute (CPSI) is to raise awareness and facilitate the implementation of ideas and best practices to inspire extraordinary improvement in patient safety and quality for all Canadians. The CPSI develops evidence-based tools and resources for governments, health organizations, leaders and healthcare providers to learn from, apply and improve the quality of care for patients, residents and clients. CPSI selects members for its Canadian Network for Simulation in Healthcare from health professionals, educators, administrators, regulators and policy makers across Canada, based on their ability to act on behalf of the entire simulation community, rather than as representatives of their respective organizations. The purpose of the group is to provide a Canadian structure for coordinating simulation efforts, and to promote simulation as an important way to educate interdisciplinary health teams in a multidisciplinary environment. Specifically, their reported objectives are to:

• Develop and foster relationships among simulation stakeholders.
• Build capacity in the simulation community.
• Develop Canadian guidelines for simulation-based practice, education and research.
• Facilitate exchange of knowledge about patient-centred simulation.
• Build the case to increase the scope and appropriate use of patient-centred simulation.
• Build the network of relationships with Canadian simulation stakeholders.

- Fine-tune the Simulation Centre Registry and Community of Practice service offerings.
- Examine simulation techniques and tools to determine their use in teaching and enhancing non-technical skills.
- Enhance effective and appropriate uses of simulation education, and identify and build a repository of Canadian best practice.
- Build on existing knowledge to develop and promote standards in patient simulation that can be used to support accreditation, programme development and research.

In this situation, some of the network's stated objectives align with the CPSI mission; however, others relate to the promotion of optimal simulation-based practices and development of a resources network to support the growth and development of the simulation community itself, not specifically related to patient safety [7].

Association of american medical colleges: simulation in academic medicine special interest group

The Association of American Medical Colleges (AAMC) represents the 161 accredited medical schools in the USA and Canada; close to 400 major teaching hospitals and health systems, including 51 Department of Veterans' Affairs medical centres; and almost 90 academic and scientific societies. AAMC's mission is to improve the health of all through serving and leading the academic medicine community. The AAMC Simulation in Academic Medicine Special Interest Group (SAM-SIG) aims to improve learning and patient care through the effective use of simulation modalities, including patient mannequins, serious gaming, virtual reality and standardized patients. Its mission is to create a community of medical schools and teaching hospitals intended to share strategies for understanding and implementing the effective use of simulation across the continuum of learning in medical education. SAM-SIG also studies the operational and business aspects of building sustainable, immersive learning environments designed to improve patient and community health outcomes. Here, the objectives of SAM-SIG focus on the application and integration of simulation technologies to improve learning opportunities for physicians and trainees that transfer to the provision of high-quality and safe patient care. This is one subset of the overarching mission of AAMC. However, like the CPSI Network,

SAM-SIG has objectives that focus on the development and maintenance of a resource network within the simulation community itself [8].

Society of academic emergency medicine: simulation academy

The focus of the Society for Academic Emergency Medicine (SAEM) is to improve the provision of care for acutely ill and injured patients through research and education. The membership of SAEM includes individuals from the field of emergency medicine with advanced degrees (e.g. MD, DO, PhD, PharmD, DSc etc.) who hold a university appointment or are actively involved in emergency medicine education or research. Other health professionals and students in a healthcare field are eligible for associate membership. SAEM advocates for health policy changes through community forums, publications, interorganizational collaborations, policy development and consultation services for physicians, teachers, researchers and students. The organization ascribes to excellence and leadership in academic emergency medicine that includes the idealism of healthcare quality, supportive camaraderie and diversity among members, and symbiotic relationships with other organizations. The SAEM Simulation Academy focuses on the development and use of simulation in emergency medicine education, research and patient care. It maintains strong ties and shares many members with the Society for Simulation in Healthcare Emergency Medicine Interest Group. As promoted on its website, the SAEM Simulation Academy's mission is to:

- Serve as a unified voice for emergency medicine on issues of simulation in education, research and patient care.
- Provide a forum for emergency medicine providers interested in simulation to communicate, share ideas and generate solutions to common problems.
- Further a coherent research mission in the various applications of simulation.
- Encourage the professional development and career satisfaction of emergency physicians involved with simulation in their academic careers.
- Foster relationships with other organizations in order to promote the use of simulation.

Like the earlier examples, the SAEM Simulation Academy focuses on the uses of simulation as they relate to the omnibus objectives of the parent organization and to facilitating a network for emergency medicine professionals interested in the uses of simulation in their practice. Of note is the explicit objective of the SAEM Simulation Academy to collaborate with other organizations whose primary mission is the use of healthcare simulation [9].

Managing emergencies in paediatric anaesthesia (MEPA)

The Managing Emergencies in Paediatric Anaesthesia (MEPA) community was formed in 2005 by the vision of Dr Matthew Molyneux, a trainee anaesthetist in Bristol, UK [10]. The objective was to create the opportunity for fellow anaesthetic trainee doctors to develop management strategies for emergencies in paediatric anaesthesia, before going on to an on-call rota with senior doctors up to 30 minutes away [10]. Where many course designers would have used the evidence base to create their own local course, the strategy employed was to engage senior representatives from all of the UK's major children's hospitals to develop a collaborative venture. Ten years on, the MEPA collaboration has 53 centres to date, in 11 countries on four continents, providing free educational interventions for both paediatric anaesthetic trainees and consultants. The shared resources provided include an evidence-based library of mapped-out simulation scenarios, with literature reviews and presentations, a training outreach system, a peer review process and a quality management framework.

Single-disciplinary healthcare simulation societies

There are advantages to professionals meeting with peers in their specific disciplines, and the rapid expansion of healthcare simulation has led to the growth of professional societies that focus solely on the uses of simulation within a single discipline. Single-disciplinary simulation societies support the development and integration of simulation-based practices within their respective disciplines, including the acquisition and maintenance of individual and team performance competencies in their domains. We will provide examples of three single-discipline healthcare simulation societies.

Association of standardized patient educators (ASPE)

The Association of Standardized Patient Educators (ASPE) describes itself as a professional association that fosters the promotion of best practices, emerging trends and scholarship in the field of human simulation and standardized patient (SP) methodology.

An international group, ASPE is dedicated to the mission of:

- Promoting best practices in the application of SP methodology for education, assessment and research.
- Fostering the dissemination of research and scholarship in the field of SP methodology.
- Advancing the professional knowledge and skills of its members.
- Transforming professional performance through the power of human interaction.

As an association with a specific focus on standardized patient methodology, ASPE provide further specialization to its membership through SIGs focusing on areas such as hybrid simulation, interprofessional education and the use of SP outside the health arena.

ASPE promotes the benefits of membership as access to resources designed exclusively for educators and others who are responsible for the design, implementation and administration of human-based simulation activities; discounts on conference fees; networking with an international multiprofessional community of interest; and the opportunity to develop leadership skills and professional growth, to name but a few [11].

International nursing association for clinical simulation and learning (INACSL)

The mission of the International Nursing Association for Clinical Simulation and Learning (INACSL) is to promote research and disseminate evidence-based practice standards for clinical simulation methodologies and learning environments [12]. INACSL promotes leadership for nursing simulation and works collaboratively with other nursing organizations, including the National League for Nursing (NLN), which is the oldest nursing education membership association in the United States [13]. The association developed the first standards for simulation practice, including INACSL Standards of Best Practice: Simulation; Simulation-Enhanced Inter-professional Education; and Simulation Design.

INACSL provides member benefits in a variety of areas, including access to the peer-reviewed journal *Clinical Simulation in Nursing*; topical educational webinars; grant opportunities to support simulation research and projects; quarterly e-newsletters; online libraries of resources; a membership directory; and opportunities to participate in formal and informal mentorship relationships. The association's LinkedIn network facilitates member connectivity; provides a venue for discussions, asking questions and sharing tips; and registers employment opportunities. INACSL sponsors an annual meeting to bring its members together with other healthcare professionals dedicated to learning and sharing information about the uses of simulation in nursing.

International pediatric simulation society (IPSS)

The International Pediatric Simulation Society (IPSS) is dedicated entirely to paediatric, perinatal and associated healthcare providers and organizations utilizing simulation-based education to improve care and safety for children. This global organization aims both to reflect and to empower the paediatric and perinatal community, through the development of a sustainable community of practice dedicated to education, research and advocacy. With a unique focus on paediatric and perinatal healthcare, the organization supports effective, safe and efficient individual, team and system improvements. The vision of IPSS is to provide optimal healthcare for children and families through simulation, championing solutions in all resource settings, complementing and enhancing the efforts of other organizations.

Gathering of healthcare simulation technology specialists (SimGHOSTS)

SimGHOSTS is an organization that supports an international population of professionals who operate medical simulation technology and manage the environments in which healthcare simulation is facilitated. In an effort to further its mission of providing educational support to healthcare simulation technologists and operations professionals, SimGHOSTS maintains affiliations with other healthcare simulation associations around the world. It hosts hands-on training events, develops and shares online resources and encourages greater community awareness through collaborative engagement. The organization provides access to discussion forums, a document database, video library and professional development activities that are accessible to members irrespective of their geographical location [14].

Multidisciplinary healthcare simulation societies

We previously described how healthcare simulation comprises activities, products and services generated and used by multiple professional disciplines (e.g. clinicians, engineers, social scientists etc.). As there are advantages to professionals meeting to advance their discipline's field of interest, so too are there advantages to assembling multidisciplinary professionals to advance the science of healthcare simulation. Professional societies that focus on healthcare simulation as it relates to multiple disciplines facilitate the types of synergistic exchanges that stimulate innovation, as well as the transfer of successful applications from one domain to another. Multidisciplinary professional societies also support the development and integration of professional practices that advance team performance competencies, especially in healthcare, where clinical practice is largely performed by interprofessional teams with diverse backgrounds and professional focuses. We will describe several multidisciplinary healthcare simulation societies, each of which centres around a common charter (i.e. geography), but maintains an interdisciplinary foundation for membership.

Australian society of simulation in healthcare (ASSH)

The Australian Society of Simulation in Healthcare (ASSH) has a mission to promote simulation education, training and research to enhance safety and quality in healthcare. ASSH represents a cross-section of the Australasian healthcare community who share a common interest in the uses of simulation for training, education, assessment, evaluation and research. Members include healthcare professionals, academics, industry groups and policy makers. ASSH provides exclusive benefits to members, such as discounted rates for professional development activities including seminars and conferences; access to online research papers; and affiliate membership with organizations such as the Society for Simulation in Healthcare (SSH) [15].

ASSH functions under the auspices of Simulation Australasia (SimAust), the peak association for the simulation community on the continent, and aims to be recognized as such by relevant decision makers in government, business and education. With numerous specialist communities such as defence, emergency management and national security, transport, resources and infrastructure, human dimensions in simulation and modelling and decision support, whose goal it is to deliver specific services to the members of the community within a specific field of practice and area of interest, members of ASSH have the opportunity to connect with simulation-focused professionals from other industries.

Society in europe for simulation applied to medicine (SESAM)

The members of the Society in Europe for Simulation Applied to Medicine (SESAM) have a wide and varied background within healthcare and medical education, all with a shared interest in and passion for medical simulation. The mission of SESAM is to encourage and support the use of simulation in healthcare for the purposes of training and research, including:

- Development and application of simulation in education, research and quality management in medicine and healthcare.
- Facilitation, exchange and improvement of the technology and knowledge throughout Europe.
- Establishment of combined research facilities.

SESAM members include individuals, legal bodies, institutions and corporations that are actively involved with the issues of simulation, or with the practical execution of simulation in the areas of education, training and research. An aim of SESAM's international initiative is to exchange experiences and reflect on how the different European simulation societies are organized, financed and structured, and which professions are represented within the respective countries. Issues that it addresses include:

- Discussing the possibility of a European medical simulation, nursing simulation and/or interprofessional simulation curriculum.
- SESAM/European Union (EU) certification of clinical skills and simulation centres in accordance with EU societies, and whether instructor certification may remain a national priority.

- How to position a society in terms of providing insights to patients and professionals in health, such as the 'Quality Label for Validated Games'.

Another aim is to increase efficiency by collaborating to create joint projects and shared activities in many EU countries, where partnerships can create a larger pool of opportunities and a stronger lobbying organization of EU politicians [16].

Society for simulation in healthcare (SSH)

The Society for Simulation in Healthcare (SSH) is a leading interprofessional society that advances the application of simulation in healthcare through global engagement [17]. SSH seeks to improve performance and reduce errors in patient care through the application of simulation-based modalities such as human patient simulators, virtual reality, standardized patients and task trainers. SSH members include physicians, nurses, allied health professionals, paramedical personnel, researchers, educators, operations specialists, computer scientists, engineers, government representatives, developers and industry partners from around the globe. SSH promotes improvements in simulation technology, educational methods, practitioner assessment and patient safety to promote the high-quality delivery of healthcare. SSH was the first simulation society to establish an accreditation programme recognizing best practices in interdisciplinary healthcare simulation. It also developed and maintains a certification programme that confers three credentialling certificates: Certified Healthcare Simulation Educator (CHSE), Certified Healthcare Simulation Educator – Advanced (CHSE-A) and Certified Healthcare Simulation Operations Specialist (CHSOS).

SSH provides numerous member benefits, including access to the impact-factored, peer-reviewed journal *Simulation in Healthcare*; educational webinars; research grants; monthly newsletters; online resource libraries; a membership directory; a mentorship programme; discussion forums; employment announcements; short courses and seminars; workshops; and discounted membership alternatives for affiliate organizations.

SSH is widely known globally, with accredited simulation programmes and 21 affiliate professional organizations on five continents. SSH maintains ties with other organizations interested in patient simulation, and partnerships with industry and small businesses engaged in the design, development and sale of simulation technology for healthcare applications. SSH sponsors an annual International Meeting for Simulation in Healthcare (IMSH), a major venue for advancing simulation in healthcare that is attended by several thousand professionals and vendors from multiple disciplines and specialisms across the globe. SSH also co-sponsors the bi-annual Asia-Pacific Meeting for Simulation in Healthcare (APMSH) and regional meetings for simulation operations professionals (SimOps).

Regional groups and alliances

Geographical distribution has also led to the formation of regional alliances, groups or guilds that serve a similar purpose to the national and international organizations, but with a focus on the needs of the local community. Examples of these types of groups include the Victorian Simulation Alliance in Victoria, Australia and the California Simulation Alliance and Florida Healthcare Simulation Alliance in the USA.

The Victorian Simulation Alliance supports the ongoing development and implementation of simulation within health professional education by fostering collegiality, collaboration, networking and sharing among those engaged in health professions education and research across the state of Victoria [18].

The California Simulation Alliance is a virtual alliance associated with the California Institute for Nursing & Health Care (CINHC). The alliance is intended to provide a cohesive voice for healthcare education in California and to benefit all simulation users in the state. Among the common benefits of these types of associations, members also have access to preferred vendor pricing agreements [19].

The Florida Healthcare Simulation Alliance (FHSA) is a central collaborative force of healthcare and other professionals creating a model for state-wide cooperation aimed at fostering uses of simulation-based practices to transform healthcare education and improve the quality and safety of healthcare delivery for all Floridians. FHSA was established through a BlueCross/BlueShield Foundation grant awarded to the Florida Center for Nursing, and now includes partnerships with academia, industry, government and health services providers throughout the state [20].

The North West Simulation Education Network (NWSEN) in the UK was created in 2010 supported by a regional health authority [21]. The health authority had previously funded a host of solitary simulation education projects and simulator hardware across a geographical area of over 14,000 square kilometres, encompassing 50 National Health Service organizations (hospitals) and 10 universities.

Many members of these types of regional simulation societies also participate in national and international societies. However, some members of the regional groups are only interested in participating at the local and regional levels. These societies provide great opportunities for addressing specific needs within a region, determining consensus agendas for action, programme planning, cooperative agreements associated with resource sharing and strategic relationships designed to advance the practices of simulation science where they are most efficacious in the respective communities. They also provide an opportunity for healthcare and other professionals to learn about healthcare simulation before investing in the larger organizations, which, despite their respective efforts to reduce barriers to engagement, may be intimidating for novice and naive users.

A theoretical perspective

It helps to understand better the development and role of these organizations if we use some theoretical perspectives derived from the field of educational anthropology, using the concept of 'communities of practice'. As Wenger et al. note: 'Communities of practice are groups of people who share a concern or a passion for something they do and learn how to do it better as they interact regularly' [22].

Lave and Wenger have provided a social anthropological viewpoint of how as humans we engage in a process of collective learning in a shared domain of human endeavour, for example engineers working on a suspension bridge or a tribe hunting together [22–26]. The term 'community of practice' was developed to explain the concept of a dynamic, alive curriculum for any learner while studying the complex social interactions occurring during apprenticeship as a learning model. The social anthropology lens focused on artificial intelligence, but latterly the concept of communities of practice is especially well suited to exploring life-long learning in healthcare, particularly as a socioconstructive interactive approach in the workplace. It is of note that many industries outside healthcare have cultivated the concept and enactment of communities of practice as a quality improvement mechanism. Ethnographical studies have highlighted how communities of practice provide meaning to knowledge capital, contribute to professional identity, develop organizational memory and legitimize participation from both experts and those aspiring to become experts [22–26].

Key elements of communities of practice

Wenger describes three key elements that are integral to all communities of practice: *the domain*, the *practice* and the *community*.

The domain constitutes an explicit learning need that all members of the community share and indeed brings the members together to form their community. With respect to discipline-specific professional communities, there is a joint recognition of the responsibility of the practitioners of the discipline to be able to maintain and develop their specific practice; for example, to better manage acute emergencies or crises that may occur while anaesthetizing children. There is also the recognition that this learning must be both sustained as career-long learning and passed on to newcomer practitioners. The domain of simulation-specific communities – whether regional or global in nature – is the provision of simulation-based education to healthcare professionals of all disciplines. These organizations have a considerably broader church of participants, particularly when one considers the spectrum of educational resources encapsulated by the term 'simulation-based education'. It is evident that members of simulation-specific communities are brought together by a learning need that they all share. However, the complexity of this need becomes more apparent as we go on to consider the relative rationales and drivers for member participation.

The practice relates to the productivity of each community in terms of collective resources created by the interactions of members. Discipline-specific professional collaborations utilize the collective expertise of members to create educational interventions using simulation techniques and technologies. These may take the form of evidence-based simulations to provide the opportunity to learn and hone the knowledge, skills, values and behaviours to manage emergencies, unique

and rare events or crisis situations. However, it may also evolve into sharing resources on how to debrief learners, mentor and set up new satellite sites of practice, promote quality-managed educational governance and perform research. Most of the simulation-specific professional societies have created resources to increase the capacity of simulation provision, the availability of or access to high-quality simulation-based education and collaboration across a large region where simulation centres or experts were already in place, but working in relative isolation. Resources include educational courses to develop faculty to teach simulation, a quality improvement framework and multimedia communication.

The community, as described by Wenger, relates to how the collective learning becomes a bond among members over time. This includes the relationship between those very experienced members and newcomers and those who interact at any opportunity as well as those who may observe only from a distance. Over time close bonds may develop between the members of all types of healthcare simulation communities. However, the presence of members at varying stages of development of their practice and the potential for competition between members for limited pooled financial support may contribute to different dynamic bonds in professional societies that are not always positively productive.

Dimensions

A community of practice has three dimensions: mutual engagement, joint enterprise and shared resources [22]. The dimension of mutual engagement encompasses a number of concepts and activities evident in all types of healthcare simulation societies. This extends beyond the opportunities provided by each for regular interactions at meetings, and relates more to legitimizing participation with equal access and equitable progression in the community. The concept is that by engaging with each other there is ownership, and in essence members become stewards shaping how their community develops. Stewardship is very evident in the collaboration among group members, with a strong focus on maintaining high-quality and creditable courses. The focus is to align with other communities to enhance the uptake of membership, promote collaboration, mentor newcomers and yet maintain credibility. The mutual engagement displayed by each community's membership takes a different form; there is membership and ownership, although this could be argued to be more distributive. Each member or centre has their own agenda and internal targets with checks and balances to meet. To explore this further, we need to appreciate the rationale for participation in each community, as discussed below.

Another dimension for consideration is that of joint enterprise. Collaboration within discipline-specific professional societies may have clear goals, as well as communication vehicles and governance structures to facilitate the achievement of these goals. The mission statement of a between-organization collaboration may, for example, focus on the provision of the opportunity to learn how to accomplish some form of simulation-centred objective, for instance using high-fidelity simulation. On the other hand, the goal of a simulation-specific professional society may be to increase the capacity for and the availability of high-quality collaborative simulation-based education across a geographical region, be it local or global. As fitting the missions of these types of societies, discipline simulation groups are typically less structured, whereas the governance structure of simulation-specific professional societies are mostly quite deliberate, with formal boards of directors, executive officers and executive staff.

The final dimension of a community of practice is shared resources. This encompasses shared terminology or language and products or resources. By and large, all types of healthcare simulation professional groups address the creation, development and distribution of new resources; however, the focus of these resources and accessibility to healthcare simulation communities may vary depending on the mission of the society. International simulation-specific societies with a global perspective may require a longer timeline to develop and share resources than is required to develop a shared library targeting a regional faculty development course in a discipline-specific simulation special interest group. However, the resources developed for regional or discipline-specific applications have enormous value for the global simulation community, and can be facilitated by the professional societies with a global mission.

Potential benefits of participation

There are a number of advantages to a collaborative healthcare community approach, particularly with respect to simulation-based education. One obvious benefit is cost-effectiveness, both financial and in terms of time investment when one considers mini-mizing the repetition of designing the same courses. The development of a cohesive quality management system that promotes the benchmarking and mainte-nance of high-quality educational provision is another. Finally in this context, the ability to target resources to research key questions across a number of sites is also advantageous.

Individuals, small groups, collaborative networks or institutions may have a plethora of reasons for participating in a community of practice. Funding to initiate or sustain the educational provision aspirations of individuals or institutions is one obvious consider-ation. Any situation where funding is dependent on participation in a community adds a clear tension to ensuring equity. However, non-participation or limited participation facilitated by support from exterior fund-ing outside the provision to the rest of the community can also be viewed as destabilizing to the social learning approach. For professional communities, funding may be necessary to ensure course provision or access to shared resources, yet this may be in direct competition with the aims of participating institutions themselves, running the courses they developed collaboratively. Organizations that can afford to run courses or have the requisite resources to run the course in their own time will flourish, whereas others in the community may not. Through the social anthropological lens of Wenger and colleagues, one can envisage members of different communities participating to build knowledge, particularly to preclude a 'reinvention of the wheel' by benefiting from shared simulation scenarios. The mainstay of the collaboration within healthcare simu-lation communities is the reuse of educational assets, the development of shared libraries and best-practice guidelines. Despite all being funded under one health authority umbrella, individuals or centres may view resources as very much 'their own' and a way to generate funds to sustain their delivery. Undoubtedly in both communities there is evidence of the mutual engagement of members to identify gaps in knowledge, innovate together and generate evidence of a return on investment for simulation education funding to benefit all of the membership. Competition in terms of pre-senting excellent research exists within most healthcare simulation communities, with strategic coordination achieved by targeted grant calls. The research output of these types of collaboration is highly valued by the membership and recognized to be mutually beneficial for all. Participating in the community to develop experience, learning directly from others by visiting and observing or participating together, is clearly evident in the many healthcare simulation professional societies. Additionally, strong mentoring elements within most healthcare simulation communities that support newcomers within the community of practice, as well as the innovation and development of broadly applicable technologies and techniques – such as trans-global tele-simulation – are also key [27].

Challenges to communities of practice

As each community targets the provision of healthcare simulation-based education, challenges related to syntax or language, consensus agreement on terminologies, establishment of technology standards and determination of best practices are points of consideration for transferable and broadly applicable implementation. This is not so much a consideration as regards buy-in for the value of healthcare simulation, but rather a challenge in determining where best practices may be determined locally, regionally, nationally or globally. Political and economic considerations, as well as workforce requirements, distribution and access to funding channels, the structural nature of healthcare systems and educational adjuncts for training clinicians, prioritization imperatives related to quality, safety and access to care, are but a few points that challenge the membership of healthcare simulation professional societies. Many simulation-focused professional groups have endeavoured to include a transparent and fair meritocracy-based network with multidisciplinary working groups for focusing on the care of patient groups, human factors and faculty development. Exercises to enhance buy-in through the adoption of Wengerian principles have greatly benefited many of these groups.

The challenges of maintaining the fidelity of the ideals of mutual engagement, joint accountability and shared resources are, as would be expected, continual in most healthcare simulation communities. Professional societies continue to grow with new membership, technology and funding opportunities, and as they do, so does the emphasis on the return on investment on both finances and the time and effort of individual members.

Economic sustainability

Healthcare is not the first industry to appreciate that a community of practice devoted to improving quality can generate value for investments. Etienne Wenger, Beverly Trayner and Maarten de Laat have created a conceptual framework both to promote and to assess the value of communities in practice [28]. The authors describe five cycles of value and data sources that can be measured both quantitatively and qualitatively. This work builds on that of Kirkpatrick [29] to explain both the complex interplays of the cycles and the integration of cycles to create value matrices for communities of practice. We have adapted each cycle to demonstrate the value of healthcare communities in the field of simulation-based education. Wenger et al.'s Cycle One is immediate value, focusing on indicators of interaction (see Table 13.1).

Cycle two is termed potential value. This relates to knowledge capital, actual and future developed by the community (see Table 13.2).

Cycle three, termed applied value, aims to capture indicators of changes in practice from varied data sources (see Table 13.3).

Wenger et al.'s fourth cycle is termed performance improvement indicators (see Table 13.4).

Table 13.1 Cycle one – immediate value: indicators of interactions.

Indicators	Data Sources
Level of participation	Attendee data, website data
Level of activity	Course/meeting frequencies Quantity of queries
Level of engagement	Intensity Challenges Continuations
Quality of interactions	Discussion of real emergencies Feedback on responses to queries
Value of participation	Feedback form Recommendations Evidence of enjoyment
Networking	Connections made
Collaborations	Joint projects Co-authorships
Reflection	Meta-conversations about community

Source: Adapted from Wenger 2011 [28].

Table 13.2 Cycle Two – Potential (future) value: Knowledge capital.

Indicators	Data Sources
Skills acquired	Self-reporting Work-based assessments Case reports
Change in perspectives	Self-reporting of attendees
Confidence	Number of difficult cases/deaths discussed Referrals
Levels of trust	Discussion of real emergencies Debates on key issues Feedback on responses to queries
Quality of output	Feedback forms Recommendations
Reputation of community	Affiliations Invitations
Production of tools to inform practice	Evaluation of products

Source: Adapted from Wenger 2011 [28].

Table 13.3 Cycle Three – Applied value: Indicators of changes in practice.

Indicators	Data Sources
Implementation of solutions	Case studies Self-reporting Incidents
Innovation in practice	New processes
Developing tools to inform practice	Research Assessment tools Debriefing tools
Reuse and evolution of products (not reinvention of wheel)	Downloads
Innovation in systems	New policies
Use of social connections	Leveraging to induce changes in practice

Source: Adapted from Wenger 2011 [28].

The fifth cycle represents the reflection on what constitutes success by the community itself (see Table 13.5). This encompasses a meta-level review of the aspirations of the community in terms of direction and vision and relationships with funders and stakeholders alike.

Table 13.4 Cycle Four – Performance improvement indicators.

Indicators	Data Sources
Participant/facilitator improvement	360-degree peer feedback Patient feedback Incident reporting
Organizational performance	Critical incident reports Serious case reviews Staff self-reporting Staff surveys Staff levels
Organizational reputation	Ability to attract staff Funding grants Patient feedback Press reporting

Source: Adapted from Wenger 2011 [28].

Table 13.5 Cycle Five – Reflection on what is success for the community.

Indicators	Data Sources
Community aspirations	New learning agenda or vision
Assessments	New metrics
Relationships and expectations	With institutions, funders and stakeholders

Finally, it includes the development of new metrics to continually assess the success or failure of the community.

Conclusion

There are three key elements that are integral to all communities of practice: the domain, the practice and the community. An exploration of these can provide an insight into how valuable communities of healthcare can be to provide a return on investment for all stakeholders, be they constituent members or commissioners/funders or healthcare provision strategists. The core dimensions of mutual engagement, joint enterprise and shared resources can generate great value, although an appreciation of specific drivers for participation and of the challenges to overcome to create and maintain a community is vital. In an age where justification for expenditure at an individual and organizational level is paramount, the ability to demonstrate a return on investment is invaluable. This is equally valuable to those creating new communities as it is to those already established. Effective communities of practice in healthcare can be expected to evolve as we learn more of the benefits and, moreover, more about how to measure this benefit.

Discipline-specific professional societies provide the opportunity for individuals to network and collaborate with others who have common interests in a shared domain expertise. These environments are essential for advancing the field of interest, but also for establishing professional identity and networking within a given discipline. For example, AMEE provides a community for professionals who focus on providing medical education in Europe and AAMC addresses the same group in North America. In this case the two organizations have similar missions within different geographical regions that also reflect different approaches to medical education. Each organization has a SIG that focuses on the uses of healthcare simulation in medical education, as opposed to other healthcare applications. The role that simulation plays in discipline-specific professional associations is directly related to the overall mission of the organization, which may or may not include simulation as a component. These SIGs facilitate an environment for individuals to maintain their discipline-specific professional identity among others in their community who have an interest in how simulation connects to their professional domain. An SIG supports the networking of those with a shared professional identity and is a conduit for deliberate engagement with organizations whose primary mission is associated with healthcare simulation.

The formalization of committees and SIGs dedicated to simulation by the organizations described here, and others, signifies that their members want to address the use of simulation-based practices within their specific discipline. The advantages of SIGs in discipline-specific professional societies are that they support the social aspects of professional identity and a common contextual framework for those using simulation in a particular domain, but also the opportunity to engage others in the discipline to expand their awareness of simulation methodologies as they relate to their specific domain. The disadvantages are the potential for a restricted viewpoint on healthcare simulation, a prescribed approach to applications and uses of simulation within the discipline, and a naivety about alternative possibilities derived from the broader simulation community. There exists a risk that this 'silo' approach will not fully embrace the capacity that simulation environments offer. To the extent that SIGs engage with the broader simulation community (e.g. SAEM), this may be mitigated. Many professionals within the healthcare simulation community maintain memberships in their discipline-specific professional societies and one or more of the professional societies that focus exclusively on the uses of healthcare simulation as a multidisciplinary construct.

Single-discipline simulation societies add tremendous value by developing techniques, libraries of shared resources and best-practice guidelines for the implementation of simulation in their professional discipline. These may include local, regional, national or global considerations, as well as determination of standards targeting discipline-specific requirements. Multidisciplinary simulation societies provide a venue for all healthcare simulation professionals to collaborate on the creation, development and distribution of single-discipline derived practices, as well as to facilitate the essential proving ground for cross-disciplinary integration of best practices across specialisms and between disciplines. Multidisciplinary simulation societies also provide a channel for determining which elements of discipline-specific simulation-based practices are broadly transferable on a global scale. Additionally, by virtue of their scale, multidisciplinary simulation societies can advocate for policy and funding influence at institutional and government levels that might challenge smaller, discipline-specific focused groups. The greatest benefits to the membership of all types of healthcare simulation professional societies is for a strong collaborative mindset among all types of groups, each of which is essential for advancing the science and implementation of healthcare simulation.

References

1 Australia and New Zealand College of Anaesthetists. Resources-endorsed guidelines [cited 2 August 2015]. Available at: http://www.anzca.edu.au/resources/endorsed-guidelines
2 American College of Surgeons. Advocacy [cited 2 August 2015]. Available at: https://www.facs.org/advocacy

3 Harvey, L., Mason, S. and Ward, R. (1995) *The role of professional bodies in higher education quality monitoring*, Birmingham, Quality in Higher Education Project.

4 Academic Pediatric Association. What's new! [cited 2 August 2015]. Available at: https://academicpeds.org

5 Association of Medical Education in Europe. Welcome to AMEE [cited 2 August 2015]. Available at: https://www.amee.org

6 ACM SIGSIM. Special Interest Group (SIG) on Simulation and Modeling (SIM) [cited 2 August 2015]. Available at: http://www.acm-sigsim-mskr.org

7 CPSI/ICSP. Canadian Patient Safety Institute [cited 2 August 2015]. Available at: http://www.patientsafetyinstitute.ca

8 AAMC. Association of American Medical Colleges [cited 2 August 2015]. Available at: https://www.aamc.org

9 SAEM. Society of Academic Emergency Medicine [cited 2 August 2015]. Available at: http://www.saem.org

10 Everett, T., Ng, E. and Power, D. *The Managing Emergencies in Paediatric Anaesthesia (MEPA) simulation course – the combination of healthcare professional training, faculty development and an international multicenter validation study.* University of Toronto Faculty Development Conference, Toronto, November 2010 (poster).

11 ASPE. Association of Standardized Patient Educators [cited 2 August 2015]. Available at: http://www.aspeducators.org

12 International Nursing Association for Clinical Simulation and Learning. Welcome to INACSL [cited 11 August 2015]. Available at: http://www.inacsl.org

13 NLN. National League for Nursing [cited 11 August 2015]. Available at: http://www.nln.org

14 SimGHOSTS. The gathering of healthcare simulation technology specialists [cited 2 August 2015]. Available at: http://www.simghosts.org

15 Simulation Australasia. Australian Society for Simulation in Healthcare [cited 2 August 2015]. Available at: http://www.simulationaustralasia.com/divisions/about-assh

16 SESAM. Society in Europe for Simulation Applied to Medicine [cited 8 August 2015]. Available at: http://www.sesam-web.org

17 SSH. Society for Simulation in Healthcare [cited 8 August 2015]. Available at: http://www.ssih.org

18 VSA. Victorian Simulation Alliance [cited 11 August 2015]. Available at: http://www.vicsim.org.au

19 California Simulation Alliance. Welcome to the California Simulation Alliance [cited 11 August 2015]. Available at: https://www.californiasimulationalliance.org

20 FHSA. Florida Healthcare Simulation Alliance [cited 11 August 2015]. Available at: http://www.floridahealthsimalliance.org

21 MacKinnon, R.H. and Farrell, M. (2010) *North West NHS Simulation Education strategic plan 2010–2011*, NWSEN, Manchester.

22 Wenger, E., McDermott, R. and Snyder, W. (2002) *Cultivating communities of practice: a guide to managing knowledge*, Harvard Business School Press, Boston, MA.

23 Wenger, E. and Snyder, W. Communities of practice: the organizational frontier. *Harvard Bus Rev.* 2000;Jan–Feb:**78** (1), 139–46.

24 Wenger, E. Knowledge management as a doughnut. *Ivey Bus J.* 2004;Jan 2–8. Available at: http://iveybusinessjournal.com/publication/knowledge-management-as-a-doughnut/

25 Wenger, E. (1998) *Communities of practice: learning, meaning, and identity*, Cambridge University Press, Cambridge.

26 Wenger-Trayner, E., O'Creevy, M.F., Hutchinson, S. *et al.* (2014) *Learning in landscapes of practice*, Routledge, London.

27 Everett, T. Bould, D. Ng, E. et al. Program innovations abstract transcontinental telesimulation: the global proliferation of the Managing Emergencies in Paediatric Anaesthesia (MEPA) course. *J Soc Simul Healthc.* 2013;Dec. **8** (8) p433.

28 Wenger, E., Trayner, B. and de Laat, M. (2011) *Promoting and assessing value creation in communities and networks: a conceptual framework*, Open University of the Netherlands, Heerlen.

29 Kirkpatrick, D.L. (1994) *Evaluating training programs: the four levels*, Berrett-Koehler, San Francisco, CA.

CHAPTER 14

Faculty development in healthcare simulation

Simon Edgar, Michael Moneypenny & Alistair May

KEY MESSAGES

Impactful and sustainable faculty development programmes:

- Are educationally literate.

- Are clinically relevant to a variety of healthcare contexts.

- Are plainly operationally focused and of obvious benefit to local or national administration or healthcare management.

- Are clearly aligned to the staff and healthcare governance aspirations and challenges of local or national organizations.

- Consider both synchronous and asynchronous components to mesh with the competing demands of time-poor clinical teams.

- Are distributed in design and provide ongoing faculty support.

Overview

Faculty development is an essential component of successful simulation programmes or activities, yet it is often overlooked. Beyond purchasing appropriate equipment and fitting out learning spaces, the third pillar of success is the realization of, and support by management and staff for, initial and continuing faculty development. This section highlights strategies used across a variety of settings to ensure that faculty development is recognized at an organizational level as a mandatory component for the establishment and ongoing business of planning, delivering and evaluating simulation learning activities.

Introduction

Simulation-based education (SBE) is an effective methodology that can be employed to develop and improve performance [1]. In healthcare, simulation is widely used to:

- Safely develop competency in the novice, through the rehearsal of designed experiences.

- Allow the clinician expert to engage with rare but impactful clinical scenarios.

- Facilitate the development of high-functioning teams through in-situ systems testing or planned scenarios.

In the hands of the violin maestro a Stradivarius will transfix the audience; in the hands of a novice it will sound terrible. The same is true of SBE, where efficacy is not inherent within the physical environment, equipment or technology being used. Instead, the activities and attributes of educational faculty associated with the planning and delivery of high-quality simulation are based on learned skills [2].

Faculty development has been described as a 'range of activities that institutions use to renew or assist faculty in their roles' [3]. Therefore, the goal of a faculty development programme in a simulation context must be to nurture its faculty so that they might make best use of whatever mode of simulation they are employing. Reviews of the literature have highlighted the importance of debriefing as a key part of faculty development programmes. However, a faculty should be skilled in all aspects of simulation, from instructional design all the way through to evaluation of impact. Still, there remains limited published work to describe the other key components and organizational infrastructure

---

Healthcare Simulation Education: Evidence, Theory and Practice, First Edition.
Edited by Debra Nestel, Michelle Kelly, Brian Jolly and Marcus Watson.
© 2018 John Wiley & Sons Ltd. Published 2018 by John Wiley & Sons Ltd.

needed to support a valid and impactful programme of development.

This chapter will give focus to the current evidence supporting the ideas and concepts of how to achieve and deliver a high-quality faculty development programme, along with commentary from the authors' own experiences. From the original BEME review [2] to recent focused reviews on the pivotal role of debriefing in faculty programmes [4], examples of successful models from around the world will be referenced, as well as some specific worked examples from the national programme in Scotland. This will sit alongside illustrations of strategies used to ensure that faculty development is recognized as an indispensable component for the establishment and ongoing business of planning, delivering and evaluating simulation learning activities.

The case for faculty development

As we have alluded to in the introduction, the delivery of efficient and efficacious interventions using simulation as a methodology requires an educational faculty trained specifically in this approach, ideally within an ongoing development and quality management infrastructure. In the authors' experience, developing and maintaining a high-quality, skilled and active simulation faculty results in individuals who act as catalysts, supporting positive change in their clinical workplace.

Healthcare simulation has evolved in many cases from unplanned purchasing of simulation mannequins, which often remained in their box for the majority of their 'life', to an era of coordinated clinical educator enthusiasm. The modern educator is keen and enthusiastic, desiring to free the caged mannequins and use 'them' for all manner of educational activities: team training, development of competency, testing of competency, rehearsal of uncommon incidents, assessment of performance, testing of clinical systems and so on. Whereas the former situation was challenging from a resource waste and underuse perspective, this new-found enthusiasm, without support for the novice faculty, can result in misuse through educational inexperience, leading to psychological harm and disengagement [5].

Within the broad spectrum of uses of clinical simulation, feedback (including debriefing) has been identified as the most important feature [2]. This requires a skilled, trained faculty capable of applying a known and rehearsed model of debriefing to the simulated event. However, in addition to the debriefing skills that are more obvious to new faculty, using simulation for planned learning requires individuals capable of meticulous application of 'constructive alignment' [6]. This means that the teacher aligns the teaching and assessment methods with the learning activities. In simulation this translates as meticulous attention to intervention design, running and debriefing in order to align it with the learning objectives.

Most simulation debriefing methods require a trained facilitator capable of constructing and maintaining a safe learning environment, managing the learning needs and personalities of the participant group, and bringing structure and direction to the conversation [7]. When simulation is employed for a specific use, the faculty will need particular knowledge and skills to optimize the activity in terms of efficacy and efficiency. For example, using simulation for complex system testing and developing of team performance in a clinical setting requires a faculty competent not solely in running immersive 'high-fidelity' and debrief-rich simulation, but also in methods such as process mapping, failure mode and effects analysis (FMEA) and table-top simulation. Equally, when employing simulation for assessment, faculty will require a clear understanding of or access to expertise relating to activity validation and assessment methodology.

From the instructional design literature [8–10] and the authors' experiences, the ideal faculty development programme appears to be one consisting of graded, periodic interventions to provide ongoing longitudinal support aligned to a form of governance with overarching quality management. Programmes perceived to be of high educational value need to be:
- Educationally literate – based on evidence and supported by expertise.
- Clinically relevant – lessons learned applicable in varied healthcare contexts.
- Operationally focused – of obvious benefit to the administration and acknowledging of challenges in healthcare management.
- Aligned to the staff and healthcare governance aspirations and challenges of host organizations.

In the next section we will consider how this can be achieved.

Structure and components of an effective faculty development programme

In the broader context of medical education, reviews of faculty development programmes describe a spectrum of structures, activities and interventions, including workshops, seminar series (both face to face and web based), time-bound courses, longitudinal programmes (e.g. fellowships) and individualized feedback [11, 12]. The use of experiential learning, provision of feedback, development and support of effective peer relationships and diversity of educational methods represent some of the key features of effective faculty development activities [12]. Equally, the diverse origins of, and populations comprising, the recipients of faculty development suggest that a 'one-size-fits-all' model will be neither acceptable nor impactful. Faculty development therefore must not only be of high quality, but also adaptable to the context in which it is being deployed.

Let us consider what structures currently exist as exemplars or may be considered to support these components.

Delivery of the faculty development programme

A superlative syllabus is not effective if it fails to reach the desired audience. Therefore, before we consider the content of a faculty development programme, we must first address the mechanisms of delivery. Ultimately, these will be determined by local factors such as geographical distribution, time allocated and resources available. The following broad principles may be helpful:

- Delivery of the faculty development programme cannot be purely a one-way channel of communication, such as a 'how to' guide distributed to all potential faculty.
- Some face-to-face component is desirable. Observing expert faculty facilitating a debriefing allows novice faculty the opportunity to appreciate the subtle techniques employed by the former in ensuring an effective debriefing. In addition, being observed by expert faculty gives novice faculty the opportunity to receive immediate feedback on their performance. Although expert faculty can provide feedback on recorded debriefing, evidence from other areas

would suggest that immediate feedback is more powerful [13].

- There are numerous ways of delivering educational content and space constraints do not allow us to review the pros and cons of each. However, the 'mastery learning' work of Barsuk et al. and McGaghie et al. [14, 15] has shown the benefit of a baseline assessment followed by deliberate practice with feedback. This model of competence progression could easily be applied to developing faculty.
- In order to make any face-to-face component as effective as possible, it is useful to consider what material can be front-loaded and made available in the weeks preceding the meeting. One must remain aware that some participants will not be motivated to engage with this material.

Delivery examples

- *SCSC^{HF} (Scottish Centre for Simulation and Clinical Human Factors).* Delivery of the initial aspects of the SCSC^{HF} faculty development programme occurs at a face-to-face two-day course held at the national simulation centre and on a mobile unit, which tours the Highlands and Islands of Scotland.
- *MSR (Israel Center for Medical Simulation):* The MSR's introductory faculty development programme is run at the Israel Center for Medical Simulation. It also offers to run workshops at other facilities.
- *BMSC (Bristol Medical Simulation Centre):* BMSC runs a two-day faculty development programme 'training the trainers' at its centre.
- *CMS (Boston Center for Medical Simulation):* CMS runs workshops at its headquarters in Boston, MA and at other host sites around the world (e.g. Spain, Colombia, Chile). It also offers an online workshop covering the Debriefing Assessment for Simulation in Healthcare (DASH) evaluation tool.
- *NHET-Sim (National Health Education and Training in Simulation):* This Australian government-sponsored training programme offers a comprehensive online training package of modules and aligned country-wide and state-delivered workshops.

Who are the participants?

Faculty composition can present a challenge to an effective faculty development programme. Simulation faculty members often have a diverse educational background and professional clinical governance structure.

Some may have no qualifications or registrations, while others may have postgraduate degrees and be subject to guidance from professional bodies, such as a nursing or medical council. In addition, the use of simulation in healthcare is widespread and in some places has been established for many years. This means that although there are many novices, there are also many experienced, although not necessarily expert, faculty members. The mechanism of delivery must therefore be able to seek out, engage and motivate a variety of faculty.

The first challenge lies in motivating and engaging people with faculty development. How a planned programme is structured must first attend to this question of 'why'. Continuing professional development (CPD) aligned to healthcare professional practice is well regulated and provided for in most countries, but the same is usually not true for simulation.

Of equal importance to consider is that many of the best educators are also busy clinicians, and implementing a robust faculty development programme with various mandatory activities may run the risk of losing talented educators [4]. That said, considering the cohort of legacy talent, while attempting to develop that future talent pool and raising the educational bar for all, is a laudable aim. It is therefore useful to have an obvious and easily accessible entry point into simulation faculty development. This acts as an induction for the simulation-naive and also 'resets the clock' for people who have been using simulation but not necessarily staying up to date with current best practice. This entry point could be either an assessment or, more engagingly, a baseline course.

Individuals also respond to incentives. In the context of faculty development this could take the form of access to national or international simulation experts, a simulation centre specialist library of scenarios or even sharing of resources (staff, equipment and material, for example). People may require skills and certification for another part of their professional practice and if the development programme can be aligned to the relevant professional frameworks, there is a clear link and motivator for potential faculty.

Participation examples

- *SCSC^{HF}:* The SCSC^{HF} accepts all types of healthcare professionals into its faculty development programme and is demand led. The typical introductory course

consists of a range of participants, although specific courses are run for teams such as the Emergency Medical Retrieval Service.
- *NHETSim:* This Australian faculty development programme's target was an impressive 4595 completions, with the aim of engaging multiprofessional learners participating or interested in simulation-based educational activity.
- *Royal College of Emergency Medicine (RCEM):* The UK-based RCEM focuses on the development of emergency medicine trainees. As an example of mandatory participation, all consultants who wish to deliver college-approved courses must attend the RCEM two-day faculty training course.
- *STELI (Simulation and Technology Enhanced Learning Initiative):* This UK initiative [16] promoted a rollout of simulation funding to support the purchase of equipment and developing infrastructure in the London hospitals. The funding support was accompanied by an explicit statement of intent from the chief executives of each of the hospital trusts involved to support individuals and teams with time and resource to develop competence in simulation-based medical education (SBME).

Programme design: stratification of content and interventions

Stratification in SBME describes the adoption of a tiered approach of courses and content with varying 'levels' aimed at mitigating the challenges of educator heterogeneity. Stratification may also assist with the concerns of balancing the time commitment needed to attain competency and the need to grow a sufficient pool of competent educators. Instead of attempting to train all simulation educators to expert level in all components of the methodology, the programme can focus on the needs of its faculty and their learners. This phased approach is clearly more appealing to healthcare delivery managers, who must often balance the challenges of running a clinical service while permitting clinical staff to spend time away from the 'front line'.

As an example of phasing and stratification:
- Help faculty to understand the concepts of constructive alignment [6] and the importance of learning objectives.
- Let them design a scenario around learning objectives.
- Help them to edit it and run and debrief it for them.

- Help them reflect on what they created, specifically in terms of the design, as you, the expert, will have run and debriefed the scenario.
- With developing debriefing skills, once they have an understanding of debriefing strategies and a model, let them perform one part of the debriefing model under your direct supervision.
- This does not even have to be in an actual debrief. Using scripted (or unscripted real) video of scenarios and debriefing can be very useful in getting faculty to practise questioning styles and debriefing strategies.

Many of these techniques will be referenced further in other chapters. Key to this style of design is a constancy of purpose; that is, an explicit overall road map of intent by the host agency shared with faculty educators and potential development programme attendees. Breaking down the skill sets can make the process more manageable for novice faculty and more obvious for the host organization and staff as to the relevance and impact of individual components in various clinical settings.

Design examples

- *CMS (Boston):* The CMS offers two introductory instructor courses, a generic course and a course designed for interprofessional operating room teams. It then offers an advanced debriefing course for graduates of these introductory courses.
- *SCSC^{HF}:* The SCSC^{HF}, in collaboration with NHS Education Scotland (NES) and a number of other stakeholders in Scotland, has developed a National Outcomes Framework for SBE faculty development. This allows both courses and programmes to map their outcomes to three different levels of SBE: awareness, introductory and advanced [17].

Educational Governance

Individuals and organizations supporting the educational development of staff or faculty have a general responsibility to provide the most impactful learning using the least resources possible, over the shortest amount of time; that is, to be efficient and effective. With simulation it is all too easy to choose the most functional mannequin in the most realistic environment and simply recreate clinical cases.

Historically, governance within simulation-based clinical education has been sparse and usually within specific clinical education courses (e.g. Resuscitation Council life support courses). This paucity of quality

statements is due in no small part to the lack of a national or international competent authority in SBE. However, like healthcare itself, governance and assurance are fast becoming overarching principles to promote effective and efficient use of this particularly expensive resource. The belief that expertise in a clinical field translates into expertise in educating others in (or outside) that field does not hold true, and this is especially the case where simulation is concerned. With so much activity within the field of simulation-based clinical education, coupled with a relative lack of governance, helping people to engage with standards in SBE is challenging. For this reason, the authors suggest that any approach that mandates components such as specific training or credentialling will be less engaging and powerful than something that is flexible, adapting to individuals and providing internal motivation. Of course, any governance and quality assurance will employ both of these dispositions, but the balance between them is key.

As an example, the faculty development programme should detail the minimum standards required of the faculty instructors. Personnel delivering the faculty development programme should be experts in SBE and effective coaches [18]. The very best facilitators are not necessarily the best coaches, and it is therefore essential to judge their effectiveness. This may include, for example, the number of courses to be run per year and the type and amount of feedback gathered from participants and observing faculty.

Governance Examples

- *AoME (Academy of Medical Educators):* There are increasingly more examples of recommended core values and standards for individuals providing clinical education. One comprehensive example is the Professional Standards document from the UK Academy of Medical Educators [19]. This describes five domains to be evidenced by individuals as part of continuing professional development in medical education:
  - o Domain 1: Design and planning of learning
  - o Domain 2: Teaching and supporting learning
  - o Domain 3: Assessment and feedback to learners
  - o Domain 4: Educational research and evidence-based practice
  - o Domain 5: Educational management and leadership

The previous version of this document was adopted by the General Medical Council for Recognition of

Trainers as part of medical doctors' revalidation or professional licensure during a process of annual clinical appraisal. Providing evidence of development in each of the five domains will therefore become a mandatory component of maintaining the position of GMC Recognized Trainer in the UK. Although these domains do not specifically mention simulation-based education, they are of course applicable.

- *NES (NHS Education for Scotland):* Scotland has a simulation-specific National Outcomes Framework for Faculty Development, referred to earlier, which outlines the broad content that would be expected in any provision for faculty development courses or programmes within simulation. This allows any individual or organization providing faculty development to map their activity to the framework and, more importantly, for developing faculty to understand what is on offer with different providers.
- *RCEM:* As already referred to, the RCEM mandates that RCEM-approved courses need to include an instructor who has attended the RCEM instructor course. In addition, the college recommends that the instructor teaches on a minimum of two courses per year [20].
- *American Board of Anesthesiology (ABA):* The ABA runs a Maintenance of Certification in Anesthesiology (MOCA) programme that mandates that its members complete a simulation course every 10 years. The course must be attended at a center endorsed by the American Society of Anesthesiology (ASA). This process of ASA endorsement involves a fee and other evidencing of requirements such as demonstration of an effective evaluation process focused on the course, the instructors and the programme.
- *Australian and New Zealand College of Anaesthetists (ANZCA):* The ANZCA requires trainees to complete the Effective Management of Anaesthetic Crises (EMAC) course. In a similar manner to MOCA, ANZCA provides accreditation to specific centres that run the EMAC course. Accreditation includes an onsite review by a college representative to ensure that it meets the requisite standards.

Final considerations to ensure longevity and impact

Operationally Focused

The primary driver for a faculty programme must be a desire to support the development and delivery

of educational interventions resulting in a sustained improvement in the participants' knowledge and skills. The stated aim of any course or programme therefore must be to deliver high-quality educational experiences to support clinical excellence. This is the key link to convince commissioners to invest in educational programmes where the alignment of the intervention is to their benefit, focused on staff and healthcare governance principles and promoting risk management and safety principles relevant to the local clinical context.

Clinically Led

Recruiting, supporting and retaining faculty are vital for the sustainability of any programme. While reflecting on the meaning of teaching and an individual's motivation to teach, Steinert and MacDonald [21] describe five themes from physicians who teach medical students and residents. Teaching:

- Is an integral part of individual identity.
- Allows a form of repayment of former teachers for one's own training.
- Gives an opportunity to contribute to the development of the next generation.
- Enables learning for the teacher.
- Is personally energizing and gratifying.

Although this small study was within a specific group of individuals, the principles are recognizable across all educational domains. Organizations taking the time to consider how to make some or all of these components highly visible to their faculty will help in motivating them to continue engaging with and supporting educational activity.

Educationally literate

Organizations must carefully weigh the trade-off between the increased time and commitment required of their clinical educators to participate in these faculty development programmes and the impact of any intervention. The continuing development of educational standards both generically and in the domain of SBE, although in its infancy, will be the primary driver for quality improvement in simulation-based education over the next decade.

Using the educational principles outlined in this chapter and others will allow commissioners to choose wisely the high-quality interventions best aligned to their organization's needs and promote the realization and support by management and staff for initial and ongoing faculty development activity.

References

1 Gaba, D.M. (2004) The future vision of simulation in health care. *Qual Saf Health Care*, **13** (Suppl 1), i2–i10.

2 Issenberg, B.S., McGaghie, W.C., Petrusa, E.R. *et al.* (2005) Features and uses of high-fidelity medical simulations that lead to effective learning: a BEME systematic review. *Med Teach*, **27** (1), 10–28.

3 Centra, J.A. (1978) Types of faculty development programs. *J Higher Educ*, **49** (2), 151–62.

4 Cheng, A., Grant, V., Dieckmann, P. *et al.* (2015) Faculty development for simulation programs: five issues for the future of debriefing training. *Simul Healthc*, **10** (4), 217–22.

5 May, A. and Edgar, S. (2016) Developing the skills and attributes of a simulation-based healthcare educator, in *Manual of simulation in healthcare*, 2nd edn (ed. R. Riley), Oxford University Press, Oxford, pp. 65–77.

6 Biggs, J. (1996) Enhancing teaching through constructive alignment. *Higher Educ*, **32** (3), 347–64.

7 Decker, S., Fey, M., Sideras, S. *et al.* (2013) Standards of best practice: simulation standard VI: the debriefing process. *Clin Simul Nurs*, **9** (6), S26–S29.

8 LeFlore, J.L., Anderson, M., Michael, J.L. *et al.* (2007) Comparison of self-directed learning versus instructor-modeled learning during a simulated clinical experience. *Simul Healthc*, **2** (3), 170–77.

9 Savoldelli, G.L., Naik, V.N., Park, J. *et al.* (2006) Value of debriefing during simulated crisis management: oral versus video-assisted oral feedback. *Anesthesiology*, **105** (2), 279–85.

10 Van Heukelom, J.N., Begaz, T. and Treat, R. (2010) Comparison of postsimulation debriefing versus in-simulation debriefing in medical simulation. *Simul Healthc*, **5** (2), 91–7.

11 Leslie, K., Baker, L., Egan-Lee, E. *et al.* (2013) Advancing faculty development in medical education: a systematic review. *Acad Med*, **88** (7), 1038–45.

12 Steinert, Y., Mann, K., Centeno, A. *et al.* (2006) A systematic review of faculty development initiatives designed to improve teaching effectiveness in medical education: BEME Guide No. 8. *Med Teach*, **28** (6), 497–526.

13 Brydges, R., Nair, P., Ma, I. *et al.* (2012) Directed self-regulated learning versus instructor-regulated learning in simulation training. *Med Educ*, **46** (7), 648–56.

14 Barsuk, J.H., Cohen, E.R., Feinglass, J. *et al.* (2009) Use of simulation-based education to reduce catheter-related bloodstream infections. *Arch Intern Med*, **169** (15), 1420–23.

15 McGaghie, W.C., Issenberg, S.B., Cohen, E.R. *et al.* (2011) Medical education featuring mastery learning with deliberate practice can lead to better health for individuals and populations. *Acad Med*, **86** (11), e8–e9.

16 Synapse. Welcome to the Simulation and Technology-enhanced Learning Initiative (STeLI) [cited 3 February 2016]. Available at: http://www.synapse.nhs.uk/pages/public/fa043e8ebb71081c7b62093ed3af7996

17 CSMEN. Clinical Skills Managed Educational Network [cited 3 February 2016]. Available at: http://www.csmen.scot.nhs.uk/

18 Gawande A. Personal best. New Yorker Magazine. Oct 3rd 2011. Available at http://www.newyorker.com/magazine/2011/10/03/personal-best

19 Academy of Medical Educators (2014) *Professional standards*, 3rd edn, Academy of Medical Educators, Cardiff.

20 Royal College of Emergency Medicine. Simulation Training [cited 3 February 2016]. Available at: http://www.rcem.ac.uk/Training-Exams/Training/Simulation Training

21 Steinert, Y. and Macdonald, M.E. (2015) Why physicians teach: giving back by paying it forward. *Med Educ*, **49** (8), 773–82.

CHAPTER 15

Programme development and sustainability in healthcare simulation

Komal Bajaj, Michael Meguerdichian, Jessica Pohlman & Katie Walker

KEY MESSAGES

- Business cases and project plans underpin successful programmes.

- Space design, delivery location and equipment considerations are key to providing the right simulation experience for the learners.

- Simulation programmes provide political legitimacy when they are aligned to the organization's mission and vision and are responsive to organizational needs.

- Adding value, maintaining political legitimacy and nurturing operations are guiding principles towards sustainability.

- Determining appropriate metrics to measure success is necessary and requires careful consideration.

Overview

Developing a healthcare simulation programme with longevity involves mindful consideration of the many elements required to ensure that the programme is relevant for all stakeholders [1]. A well-planned programme delivers a curriculum through a range of simulation modalities, has trained and certified simulation educators and specialists (technicians), is aligned to the organization's mission and vision and is delivered in an environment where reality is maximized. The authors will describe the necessary elements of simulation programme development, the impact of the centre design and equipment considerations. A public value-creation theory and sustainability model will be presented, including governance and management considerations to ensure that programmes meet organizational goals and deliver on training objectives, while providing safe, efficient and transparent outcomes. Using this literature for simulation centre sustainability may help us better understand value in the public sector and how to measure it more effectively.

Introduction

The administration of healthcare simulation programmes is maturing as the field continues to grow. The use of business plans and project plans during development, as well as the application of public-sector business theory when addressing sustainability, are critical managerial aids to establish programmes that will flourish over time. An understanding of the external environment is key to establishing a programme where enriching collaborations can be nurtured. Being cognisant of the internal environment, where the programme resides in terms of the organizational structure and who the simulation director reports to will determine visibility and leverage for the programme. Careful consideration of programming, space utilization and equipment purchases will start the simulation centre on a stable foundation. Thinking about the programme in a way that will add value to the organization, where political legitimacy is cultivated, and one where operations are nurtured, will provide sustainability in a thoughtful way.

Development

Developing a business case and project plan

Business case and project plan development will assist both the centre director, their team and their supervisor to clearly delineate challenges as well as resources that will be required. Bartlett Ellis et al. [2] describe the headings of the business plan as including:

- Problem identification and alignment with strategic priorities
- Needs assessment
- Stakeholder analysis
- Market analysis
- Intervention implementation planning
- Financial analysis
- Outcome evaluation

A fundamental project-planning template would include a list of tasks, each with an assigned, well-described cost, timeline and personnel responsible for completion. A Gantt chart may suffice to record this information [3]. There are a plethora of business planning and project management templates online. Use a template that will meet your needs without being too complex. Some organizations have their own templates and it would be prudent to use your organization's template before looking further. Funding for simulation programmes can come through different channels, such as grant funding (both direct and indirect), budgeted line item or philanthropy, and more often is a mix of all three. Being cognisant of these different modes can help maximize the funding allocated to the simulation programme. Careful consideration of the gap the programme addresses, the faculty who will need to be trained, the curriculum developed and how the simulation experience will be deployed – at point of care, in the hospital environment or in a standalone simulation centre – will expedite the development and delivery process [4].

Programming and space considerations

Designing a simulation space is a process that requires resources, creativity, organization and attention to detail. When considering construction, there are key elements that demand attention prior to the first nail being driven in. In such a project that combines education and design, we must think about mission and vision, members of the team, centre size, movement and flow, room types and audio/visual/environmental considerations.

Mission and vision

It is important first to perform a needs assessment of the institution to determine where the resources are going to be applied. This can be achieved by identifying important stakeholders who will drive the utilization of the centre. Stakeholders should include the faculty, who will be utilizing the centre as they will be driving the curriculum and programmes. Other stakeholders to consider include the administration that holds the purse for the programme. This group will control the amount of resources available to both build and sustain a programme, and will help define its mission and vision. Having an 'if you build it, they will come' philosophy, without a mission and vision, is not likely to bear fruit. By constructing the vision of the programme, you create the core values and purpose of the simulation centre as well as a direction for its future [5]. Once you have identified your programme's needs and the deliverables, you are able to start thinking about design as part of the mission.

The team

A simulation design team must include at least project manager, architect, contractor, owner, faculty and simulation design consultants. Simulation design consultants are team members who have had previous experience with simulation education; if none is available this can be outsourced to consultants. With this team, it is important to determine what type of simulation space is going to be pursued. Will it be a mannequin-based programme? Does the institution want to create a virtual hospital? It is important to ask questions like these, relying on the mission and vision of the programme to better understand how the space can best achieve its needs [5].

Centre size

The size of the simulation space depends on many factors. First, what type of space exists at the institution? Are you retro-fitting an old space or are you building a completely new space? If you are retro-fitting the space, you may not have a choice about the dimensions of the area. If you are creating a new space, think about the number of people using the space simultaneously that the space will need to accommodate.

If you are given one room, think about the types of functions the room will need to achieve. Are you teaching 40 students central line insertion using part-task trainers? Are you teaching interdisciplinary code response teams teamwork strategies? When you are given only one room, the room needs to be modular and to adapt to the programme's educational needs.

If you are given multiple rooms, think about how each of the rooms will adapt to certain educational activities. Will you have an operating room that differs from the critical care suites already provided? Will you have clinical rooms where simulated patients perform objective structured clinical examinations? Once again, tailoring the size to the needs based on the mission and vision as well as to the faculty deliverables will guide the team towards success.

Flow

How people will move through the space during an educational activity is also important. Will your learners need to debrief in the same room where they have performed their simulation or will they move to a room next door? Is the classroom a separate area that requires a five-minute walk to get to from the simulation experience? Will the location of the bathrooms necessitate longer breaks or delays during a learning activity? Proximity of storage rooms where equipment is held will affect preparation and breakdown times. Thinking about how wide the hallway needs to be to get equipment like stretchers and storage carts through has to be part of the plan. Attention to ensuring that the facility complies with local accessibility standards should not be overlooked. Discussion with your contractor regarding the type of flooring needed to accommodate heavy traffic will avoid early maintenance.

Room types

In situations where there is more than one room, the room types will once again be defined by the requirements of the programme. Does there need to be a conference room that will have direct instruction? When considering assessment, will you need a direct observation room or will video transmission suffice? If there is an audio-visual component to the programme, will a separate room be required to house the server? Will the room need cooling? If moulage is anticipated to be a large part of your programme, will a separate prep room be dedicated to this? The control room will house your simulation operators, who will manage the magic behind the glass. As cases become more complex, attention to sound and ability to see will become more important.

Storage is an often overlooked necessity of the simulation centre. It is imperative to have a clean, dedicated and secure space to house equipment and supplies. A quarter to a third of the total space dedicated to the centre should be allocated to storage space to allow for programme growth and expansion. In addition to clinical rooms, here is a list of possible room types:

- Observation rooms
- Storage room
- Audio-visual room and/or an IT room
- Changing room/locker room
- Bathroom
- Control room
- Kitchen
- Debriefing room
- Conference room/auditorium
- Offices
- Copy room
- Preparation/moulage room
- Apartment (home care/extraction room)
- Lobby/entrance

Audio-visual/environmental considerations

Identifying whether the centre needs an audio-visual system is part of the project plan. Anticipating if faculty will want to broadcast a simulation in real time or video-record it for playback affects the range of educational strategies available. Placement of cameras and microphones needs to be pre-determined. Are you considering low-tech options such as cell-phone video or higher-tech options such as an integrated system that allows for bookmarking and more comprehensive reviewing?

Depending on the size of the centre, having different zones may help cut costs for heating and electrical. As mentioned, cooler zones for audio-visual systems may be needed, while more adjustable heat zones will be appropriate for higher-traffic areas. Ask your contractor what type of lighting and sound insulation would be best in the space.

Equipment selection considerations

Long before making equipment purchases, one must have a clear understanding of the courses and types of simulation sessions that will be conducted. The more long range you can predict, the better your equipment purchases will be. It is best to consult all stakeholders to determine what their key training needs are and that these align with the organization's mission and vision. Not all training needs can be addressed via simulation, due to either financial constraints or limitations of simulation. It is also prudent to consult with other key players in your healthcare delivery system – infection control, risk management and so on – to ensure that the equipment selected meets hospital-wide training initiatives. Finally, it is important to locate under- or unutilized equipment that may already be present in your facility. It is advantageous to collaborate with departments that have purchased such equipment – an optimal solution might be one where the simulation centre gains additional equipment that you do not need to purchase and the department can begin training on equipment that was not being optimally utilized.

Once you are clear what you will be delivering, it is time to match the best equipment to your intended simulations. It is important to think of the skill level of your learners and how they will use the equipment. Are you teaching novices, when as a result your training will almost all be procedural-based skills? Are you teaching teamwork and communication to interdisciplinary teams? Such questions will help focus your search on the various categories of equipment: partial-task trainers, full-bodied mannequins and virtual reality trainers. Furthermore, it is important to weigh up how simulated patients will be utilized within the programme and how this will affect your equipment needs.

The process of purchasing equipment can be tedious – it requires careful investigation and evaluation of various types of equipment. Price should not be the driving factor in equipment selection. It is best to spend your budget on a smaller number of carefully selected pieces of equipment that will work hard for your centre, rather than to purchase large quantities of lower-cost equipment that may not meet your needs or will not stand up to prolonged use. Identify the list of 'must have' features, as well as the 'nice to have' features from your stakeholders. Begin your research by looking for items that have all of your 'must have' features. Talk to neighbouring simulation centres and ask them what equipment they are currently using and if they would purchase that equipment again in the future. After narrowing your search down to a few good

options, invite those vendors in to demonstrate their products.

Assemble a team of stakeholders to evaluate the equipment. Members of this team should be available to evaluate all of your potential options and provide their preferences. Determine the pieces of equipment that will provide the best value to you: pieces that allow training on a multitude of skills or that can be used in a variety of applications are often the best options given the limited secure storage space that most centres have. Ensure that skills are not being duplicated in other equipment purchases. If equipment pieces are narrowly focused or address skills that are necessary but costly, see if you can make agreements with neighbouring simulation centres to purchase that equipment together and share it between the facilities.

Finally, when equipment funds are tight, determine whether you can make low-cost trainers or models yourself. Not all simulation equipment needs to be commercially purchased. Think outside the box and see if there is a way in which you can replicate the skills in a part-task trainer with items from a craft store or hardware store.

Sustainability

There are several complex factors to consider when developing strategies to ensure the ongoing sustainability of a newly created simulation programme. Dr Mark H. Moore, an authority in public management, provides a theoretical framework to help identify sources of support as well as challenges when trying to move an agenda forward [6]. The next section describes the three components of Moore's strategic triangle as illustrated in Figure 15.1 – public value, political legitimacy and operational capabilities – as well as providing practical suggestions and tools to explore these areas to find programme-sustaining solutions.

Creating public value
Value itself can have multiple dimensions, depending on its context or from whose point of view it is being ascertained. For example, Benington identifies several dimensions of value-added in the public realm, including 'economic', 'social-cultural', 'political' and 'ecological' value [7]. Furthermore, he posits that value is a 'contested concept which depends upon a

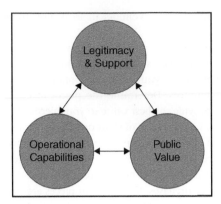

Figure 15.1 Moore's strategic triangle. Source: Reproduced with permission from Moore M. Creating Public Value: Strategic Management in Government: Harvard University Press; 1997.

deliberative process within which competing interests and perspectives can be debated' [8]. Therefore, since value greatly depends on the unique environment and challenges in which it is being discussed, being clear about what that value means to different individuals is an important first step in creating substantive value.

REFLECTIVE EXERCISE

What value does your programme create? Consider value from different stakeholders' perspectives.

For (a) your superiors, (b) your peers and (c) your trainees/other subordinates:
• What problem are you solving?
• What is your goal?
• What is your guiding message?

Cultivating political legitimacy

Political legitimacy is a vital ingredient in the survival of a simulation programme. Legitimacy can come from a variety of sources and often catalyses the actions necessary to create or maintain value.

REFLECTIVE EXERCISE

When attempting to attract the resources needed for sustainability, consider the following target areas and

list what support each may offer in advancing your mission: (a) institutional interests, (b) directives from regulatory organizations, (c) legal and ethical mandates, (d) media coverage and public relations, (e) Your professional network.

Professional social networks themselves are complex and are often the hidden avenues through which meaningful action takes place (or is undone) within organizations [9]. Networks comprise many different associations (individuals, groups, institutions) who interact for a multitude of reasons, including advice seeking, task sharing and information gathering. Recognizing the structure of your own network will help you be a more effective advocate for your agenda and circumvent challenges.

REFLECTIVE EXERCISE

When contemplating strategies to harness your professional social network, consider the following to identify important individuals/groups in your network:
• Who are the important individuals who support or block your agenda? What are their sources of power (title, expertise, network centrality, social influence, funding, other)?
• What are the important groups/organizations that support or block your agenda?
• How are these individuals and groups related?
Draw the network surrounding you and your agenda. Begin by drawing a circle in the middle of the page called 'us'. Next, place those with whom you have strong ties with a connecting line in green and those with whom you have weak ties with a connecting line in red on the page, so that people in the same organization are near each other. Use a green marker for supporters and a red pen for blockers. Finally, draw circles around people in the same organization and add any other organizations from the list of blockers and supporters you identified (again using red and green to distinguish supporters and blockers).

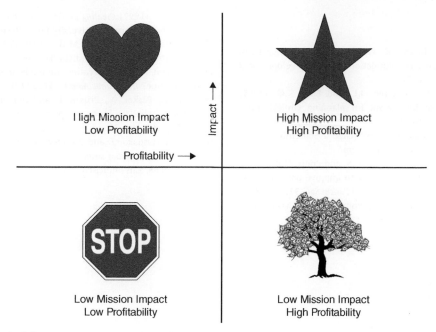

Figure 15.2 Sustainability matrix map. Source: Reproduced with permission from Bell J, Masaoka J, Zimmerman S. Nonprofit Sustainability: Making Strategic Decisions for Financial Viability: Jossey-Bass; 2010.

Nurturing operations

The first half of this chapter discusses development of a simulation programme and the critical role that vital operations play from inception to opening. Moore's triangle focuses managers on considering what operational capabilities (including innovations) the simulation programme currently relies on (or needs to develop in the future) to deliver value.

Depending on which quadrant an activity is placed in on the matrix map, a strategic imperative emerges. This helps clarify the actions that would most likely strengthen your simulation programme's value and improve the organization's sustainability.

Conclusion

The groundwork for a sustainable simulation programme is laid during its inception. This chapter has highlighted key elements that require deliberate attention during all phases of planning and execution. Every simulation programme is different depending on its mission and vision and the sector of the healthcare or education system it is serving. Consideration of space and equipment and how and where the programme will be delivered is essential. Thinking of the value the programme adds, its political legitimacy and how to nurture its operations are key to long-term success.

REFLECTIVE EXERCISE

Bell et al. [10] think of success in not-for-profit organizations as the relative impact or value of the programme versus the profitability. In Figure 15.2 is a grid where you can plot your programmes to understand more fully the value they are adding both to the organization and financially. You may decide to stop delivering programmes that fall into the lower left quadrant, for instance. Plot your existing products and services as well as initiatives that you are considering on Figure 15.2.

References

1 Seropian, M.A., Brown, K., Gavilanes, J.S. and Driggers, B. (2004) An approach to simulation program development. *J Nurs Educ.*, **43**, 170–74.

2 Bartlett Ellis, R.J., Embree, J.L. and Ellis, K.G. (2015) A business case framework for planning clinical nurse specialist-led interventions. *Clin Nurs Spec.*, **29**, 338–47.

3 Gantt. What is a Gantt chart? [cited 2 September 2016]. Available at: http://www.gantt.com/

4 Salas, E., Wilson, K.A., Burke, C.S. and Priest, H.A. (2005) Using simulation-based training to improve patient safety: what does it take? *Jt Comm J Qual Patient Saf.*, **31**, 363–71.

5 Collins JC, Porras JI. Building your company's vision. *Harvard Bus Rev.* 1996; **74**(5), Sept–Oct:65–77.

6 Moore, M. (1997) *Creating public value: strategic management in government*, Harvard University Press, Boston, MA.

7 Benington, J. and Moore, M.H. (2010) *Public value: theory and practice*, Palgrave Macmillan, London.

8 Benington, J. (2009) Creating the public in order to create public value? *Int J Public Admin.*, **32**, 232–49.

9 Cross, R., Parker, A., Prusak, L. and Borgatti, S.P. (2001) Knowing what we know: supporting knowledge creation. *Org Dyn.*, **30**, 100–20.

10 Bell, J., Masoaka, J. and Zimmerman, S. (2010) *Nonprofit sustainability: making strategic decisions for financial viability*, Jossey-Bass, San Francisco, CA.

SECTION IV
Elements of simulation practice

CHAPTER 16

Ethics of healthcare simulation

Nathan Emmerich, Gerard Gormley & Melissa McCullough

KEY MESSAGES

- Although simulation is often considered to provide a *safe* environment for experiential learning without risking harm to 'patients', we are aware that learners, and those directly involved in the learning process, are at potential risk too.

- Facilitators of simulation-based education need to continue to advance ethical frameworks around such learning.

- Such ethical frameworks should guide best practice in how risks are minimized for those who learn and benefit from such teaching practices.

- In terms of *virtue ethics*, simulation-based education can contribute to the development of a student into a professional.

- If the process of debriefing and reflection becomes merely a performative technique, simulation-based education may fail to be as beneficial for students in generating self-knowledge, and consciously realizing the process of their professional development.

Overview

Simulation-based education can provide valuable opportunities to provide learners with an insight to the many complex dimensions of real clinical practice. Although it is often considered to provide a *safe* environment for experiential learning without risking harm to 'patients', we are aware that learners, and those directly involved in the learning process, are at potential risk too. Facilitators of simulation-based education need to continue to advance ethical frameworks around such learning. Such ethical frameworks will guide best practice in how risks are minimized for those who learn and benefit from such teaching practices.

For the purposes of this chapter, ethics can be defined as the moral principles that govern a person's behaviour or the conduct of an activity. Given that the principles of biomedical ethics – autonomy, beneficence, non-maleficence and justice – continue to provide a common ethical vocabulary in the healthcare professions, these principles can lend themselves to our discussion of the ethics of simulation. We will also introduce an analysis of the ethics of reflective education and a virtue ethics, informed by a Foucauldian perspective, to examine the ethical responsibilities of healthcare educators to provide a safe learning environment that best prepares learners.

Introduction

Health and social care professional education aims to provide learners with a transformative experience so that they can offer competent, compassionate and safe healthcare as professionals. Simulation-based methods are increasingly being used to provide learning experiences for students and practitioners to advance their clinical skills and behaviours [1]. Simulation-based education is being used alongside, and as a complement to, more traditional educational methods [2–4] and, indeed, some consider its introduction to be an ethical imperative [5]. Unquestionably, simulation will continue to offer new types of learning experiences in the future as this pedagogical paradigm matures and develops.

Fundamentally, simulation-based education offers two key learning opportunities. First, it provides learners with an invaluable opportunity to 'rehearse' and incrementally advance their skills before transferring them to the clinical setting. This reduces the possibility

---

of learners harming patients unnecessarily (for example, first practising peripheral vein cannulation on a mannequin arm and then progressing to a real patient). Second, simulation can create learning opportunities that may not be readily available, or frequently occurring, in clinical practice (for example, managing a patient with a tension pneumothorax). Thus, learners can accumulate a greater level of experience than is the case were simulations not made available. Of course, such experience cannot, in the final analysis, perfectly replicate or replace encounters with real patients in clinical practice. Nevertheless, the experiences that simulation provides remain valuable and cannot be dismissed as 'mere simulation'. A key tenet of simulation is that it provides a *safe* environment for experiential learning without risking harm to *patients*.

Simulation can provide valuable opportunities to challenge learners and allow them to gain insight into not only the clinical but also the complex emotional and psychological landscapes of healthcare environments. For simulation to achieve its full pedagogical potential, it is important that such learning experiences are not overly simplistic and therefore predictable. Simulations must, to whatever degree appropriate and possible, provide sufficient challenge for individuals to learn from by replicating the complexities of clinical practice and not simply provide an opportunity for exercising technical skills. Thus, simulations should provide *desirable challenges*, such as adverse events, and opportunities to manage uncertainty and respond to the possibility of error. Simulation has the potential to allow learners to encounter and explore the boundaries of their clinical and professional competence in order that they might draw on these experiences in the interest of their future clinical and professional development. As such, simulation pedagogy offers an opportunity for students to better 'know thyself', an essential component of contemporary understanding of reflective education and practice.

However, if we consider the use of such learning experiences in more detail, the potential risks to learners can be brought into focus. Regardless of the degree of simulation complexity, learners are at risk of potential harm, both psychological and emotional, in their pursuit of best preparing themselves for providing excellence in patient care. The process of transforming students of the healthcare professions into professional practitioners is not a simple one. It is less a case of

moving from A to B than it is of moving from A to B via a number of intermediate – and not necessarily linear or incremental – steps. While simulation must stretch students, it should be carefully designed so as not to be insurmountable or overwhelming. While psychological and emotional harm can and should be anticipated in simulation-based education, strategies must be set in advance to minimize the harm but maximize the learning. Such concerns provide the primary basis of ethical concerns in simulation.

For the purposes of discussion, ethics can be defined as the moral principles that govern a person's behaviour or the conduct of an activity. Conducting simulation in the context of healthcare education should endeavour to be guided and informed by moral principles and an analysis of the risks and benefits of simulation. Beauchamp and Childress's principlism is an often-taught framework for ethical reasoning and thought in healthcare professional education [6]. Given that the principles of biomedical ethics – autonomy, beneficence, non-maleficence and justice – continue to provide a common ethical vocabulary for the healthcare professions, these principles can lend themselves to our discussion of the ethics of simulation. Nevertheless, given that the nature and practice of education differ from those of healthcare, it would be unwise to limit our discussion of the ethics of simulation to these four principles alone. Thus we also introduce an analysis of the ethics of reflective education and a virtue ethics informed by a Foucauldian perspective to our examination of the ethical responsibilities of healthcare educators to provide a safe learning environment that best prepares learners for good clinical practice [7, 8].

Benefits and risks of simulation

Simulation-based education is increasingly being used in the training of future and current health professions. Underpinning this teaching practice is a mounting evidence base that is attributing many benefits to this form of learning education: enhanced patient care, patient safety, error management and patient autonomy are many of the purported benefits of simulation [1–3, 9–11]. It should be noted that while there is a growing evidence base, some studies have shown that the effects of simulation-based training may not always transfer to the real clinical arena [12]. However, on balance and with such growing evidence of the benefits of simulation-based education, it could be argued that it would be unethical to wait for unequivocal proof to emerge in order to embrace innovative simulated-based learning initiatives where possible and practicable in clinical education [2, 5].

Although considered to be a *safe* learning environment, there are inherent risks in simulation-based education. While no *actual patients* may be harmed during a simulation-based learning activity, all individuals involved in the learning experience are at a degree of potential risk; simulation-based education is not risk free for either the learners or the role players. We might also consider the potential impact of simulation learning on future patient care.

The four principles applied to simulation

The four principles of biomedical ethics [6, 13] are in common parlance across healthcare and healthcare education – including attempts to integrate the teaching of medical ethics into simulations [14]. While they do not exhaust the ethics of healthcare education, and may not even provide the best approach to its evaluation, they do offer a collectively comprehensible starting point and one that is suitable to an introductory chapter such as this.

The principle of autonomy can be considered as the counterpart of respect for people. When designing and implementing simulations, it is important to bear in mind that one should maintain respect for all those involved. Medical education has an unfortunate history of using humiliation as a pedagogical tool. While this activity has not been entirely eliminated from medical culture, that should not be an excuse for it to appear in simulation exercises. Of course, maintaining respect for learners does not mean designing ineffectual tests or exercises in which failure is not possible. Rather, it means recognizing the range of outcomes that a simulation might produce and having appropriate responses in place to support students as their education and training progress. One might connect this to broader notions of reflective education. Prior to undertaking a simulation, students need to be briefed in what they might expect and what is expected of them. Subsequently, they need to be debriefed about their performance and about any

opportunities for further development. At this point, healthcare educators can offer students an external perspective on their performance and encourage them to reflect on this, their performance in the simulation and their learning more generally. Thus, healthcare educators can (and should) express their respect for learners through competent and comprehensive pedagogical design. Furthermore, this perspective indicates that, when expressed in the context of reflective education, the 'ethic' of respect for persons is tied to its pedagogical ethos.

Students of the healthcare professions are adults who undertake their studies autonomously. While the *transformative* nature of such education calls into question simplistic notions of informed consent – no students can fully realize the implications of their decision to undertake a professional programme of study over a number of years – it is nevertheless the case that educators should respect reflective learners as autonomous people. This means providing them with instructions, examinations and feedback that are clear and engage them as individual learners. Again, this should be taken to mean that instructions for particular simulations cannot be 'incomplete' or in some way ambiguous. Nor does it mean that feedback must be honest to the point of brutality.

The ethical imperative of respect for people is also operative in the context of simulations that include actors in the role of patients or 'expert patients'. It is important for educators to be aware that the contribution these individuals have to offer may extend beyond what educators presume or expect. Part of the purpose of involving simulated patients and actors in healthcare education is to introduce the kind of lay or patient perspective that is present in clinical practice to the professional education of healthcare students. Thus there are good pedagogical reasons to respect the contribution that external contributors make to healthcare education and simulation. This is not, of course, to suggest that such individuals need not be offered guidance on what is expected of them, or with regard to what they might expect. Rather, it is to suggest that they be allowed a certain degree of freedom to 'speak for themselves', from their own experience, and for their potential to contribute not to be restricted or constrained from the outset. Achieving a mutually consistent understanding of the responsibilities of patient actors is, one might say, a two-way street [15].

As this discussion regarding autonomy or respect for people suggests, educators should attend to their pedagogical motivations and ensure that they act beneficently and not maleficently. The education of healthcare professionals takes a number of years and, rather like medical practice, what might seem like harm in the short term is, in fact, done in the interests of the patient/student over the long term. This is true of simulation as a formative and summative approach to teaching.

Simulations can legitimately challenge and even stretch students. It is not unethical for students to experience failure, and simulations can be designed to include the unavoidable death of the patient [16]. Such experiences do not necessarily lead to emotional or psychological harm. What is of ethical importance is the way in which educators and students respond to such experiences. In practice, all medical professionals will undoubtedly experience failure at some point – they will have patients who die and patients they could have better served – thus medical education must equip students with the ability to respond to such experiences, to build on them and to do better in future. The relevant morality is akin to what Bosk called 'forgive and remember' [17]. Challenging simulations provide an opportunity to inculcate in students, both individual and collectively, the ability to respond to the inevitable experience of failure.

As simulation becomes ever more present in health and social care curricula across many institutions, there are a number of limitations to its provision: expense in terms of resourcing such activities and the expertise of facilitators [18]. In consideration of the ethics of simulation, it is important to remember equality of learner opportunity. Furthermore, institutions should pay particular attention to the level of resources allocated to simulation in clinical education [19]. It should be noted here that often variation in simulation provision across programmes of study is not easily attributable to the financial status of institutions, schools or departments. Rather, individuals leading programmes of clinical study may simply lack experience and interest. It is in terms of 'justice' not only to the students but to the patients and populations served that institutions should continue, within their finite budgets, to prioritize simulation-based activities in keeping with best practice and evidence in whatever way they can. At a minimum, however, effective and sound simulation in clinical education requires appropriate funding for training of staff – including appropriate time made available to them – and facilitators, simulated patients (recruitment and usage), equipment and other overheads to help minimize risks to learners, professional colleagues, future patients and their families. The limiting factors to successful simulation have much to do with the facilitator(s) of the simulation and include effective design, environment, pre-briefing and debriefing and facilitator adaptability during the simulation. All of these require that the facilitator has had specialized training to avoid lack of engagement and buy-in from learners and reinforcement of errors and/or inappropriate practice. Hence, the importance of prioritized funding and support from management within the organization.

Virtue ethics: building character through simulation

The arena of healthcare education involves the development – or, more accurately, the transformation or metamorphosis [20] – of students into professionals. Given the characterological dimensions of such educational programmes, we should recognize that there is an (implicit and explicit) normative purpose to their pedagogical content. In this context, we can appreciate the degree to which professional education is an apprenticeship; the degree to which it involves induction into a particular culture and way of being. In such accounts it is clear that students become professionals through a set of complex developmental processes that have impacts on them as moral individuals [21, 22].

Such views exhibit an affinity with virtue ethics, a perspective that presumes an expanded conception of 'the ethical' and, unlike mainstream approaches to applied ethics, one that facilitates a consideration of the moral psychology underpinning our actions. Thus, while virtue ethics runs counter to the prevailing norm of focusing moral judgement on 'actions' rather than 'individuals', it connects with common practice in healthcare education. For example, it is normal for applicants to medical schools to be selected on the basis of their (perceived) character, and it is common for this to be seen as the basis for future development. Furthermore, such development is not the responsibility of educators alone, but something that students are required to pursue for themselves. This is particularly true in the contemporary era, where ongoing professional development is seen as a basic requirement of practice.

The education of healthcare professionals therefore aims to instil in students a particular relation to their own, and especially professional, self; one in which they are capable of reflective monitoring and evaluating themselves in order that they might pursue and self-direct their own further development. Not only is this consistent with the medical imperative for physicians to know themselves, but there is also a particular resonance with the Foucauldian account of ethics, something that is usually understood as a contemporary, if unorthodox, form of virtue ethics [23]. Here ethics involves the care or, perhaps better, *government* of the self by the self. The particular forms this might take are essentially political, which is to say that they are inescapably shaped by social, cultural and historical forces. The conception of the 'reflective professional' and, more importantly, their education [24, 25] is suffused with what Foucault would call technologies of the self, cultural processes through which the self continually 'makes' and 'remakes' itself according to aesthetical – which is to say ethical – norms [26]. This positions healthcare education as an activity that is essentially ethical; it requires students to develop a specific relation to their own self, something that, for Foucault, is the very essence of ethics.

Simulation exists within the ecology, or normative ethos, of reflective pedagogy. Indeed, it has a particular role to play within the reflective approach to healthcare education. In the first instance, simulations provide students with the opportunity to practise – or 'dress rehearse' – their knowledge and skills at a specific point in time. This means that they can be used to structure particular courses and, correctly positioned, they can fundamentally contribute to the reflective development of healthcare students. In this view, simulations are not simply 'tests' of knowledge or abilities, but opportunities for educators and students to examine their demonstrable strengths and weaknesses, and to do so on the basis of performance that seeks to approximate to clinical practice.

As with reflective portfolios, there is a danger that simulations are reduced to the *merely* performative [27]. While there must be an element of performance in the design and completion of any simulation, part of what simulations offer students is the opportunity to practise being in the clinic through a kind of rehearsal performance. Such experiences can contribute to the formation of the relevant professional dispositions and/or habits in a manner similar to the actual accumulation of observational and practical clinical experience [28]. Thus, concern regarding performative acts that are unethical primarily pertains to the authenticity of subsequent processes of self-reflection and the accuracy with which they are reported to and discussed with both oneself, peers and others. Students are predisposed to present themselves as meeting the imagined or actual expectations of educators. The project of reflective pedagogy can be undermined by attempts to fulfil these expectations. First, students' reflective accounts might be misleading or even false; and second, the lessons that students learn by providing accounts that misrepresent their experience will run counter to the ideals that reflective education seeks to impart.

In terms of Foucault's perspective on ethics, if the process of reflection becomes subordinated or instrumentalized as a merely performative technique, it does not cease to be a technique of the self – it can still contribute to the pedagogical construction (or assembly) of the individual as a professional – but it does cease to be a way of generating self-knowledge, of students knowing themselves and consciously realizing the process of development. An authentic process of reflection can be one way to 'care for the self', but this is no longer the case if such processes become little more than expectation-meeting performances.

Conclusion

The health and social care needs of our societies are changing and will continue to change. With a rapidly expanding evidence base, ageing population and increasing number of patients living with multiple co-morbidities, healthcare provision is becoming more complex and challenging. Simulation can provide valuable opportunities to challenge learners and allow them to gain an insight into not only the clinical, but also the complex emotional, social and psychological dimensions of the real working environment. With the greater use of simulation and increasing evidence base, simulation-based educational methods will continue to open up new approaches to learning. Although often considered to provide a *safe* environment for experiential learning without risking harm to *patients*, we are aware that learners, and those directly involved in the learning process, are at potential risk. Given the emphasis on the sociomaterial aspects of simulation, material modifications are often made to greatly reduce, but not totally mitigate, physical risks. However, simulation has the potential also to cause significant psychological and emotional harm. Facilitators of simulation-based education will need to continue to advance ethical frameworks around such learning. Such ethical frameworks will guide best practice in how risks are minimized to those who learn and benefit from such teaching practices. While simulation-based learning aims to reduce harm to actual patients, harming learners is also of benefit to no one.

References

1 Cook, D.A., Hatala, R., Brydges, R. *et al.* (2011) Technology-enhanced simulation for health professions education: a systematic review and meta-analysis. *JAMA*, **306** (9), 978–88.

2 Gaba, D.M. (2004) The future vision of simulation in health care. *Qual Saf Health Care*, **13** (suppl 1), i2–i10.

3 Issenberg, S.B., McGaghie, W.C., Petrusa, E.R. *et al.* (2005) Features and uses of high-fidelity medical simulations that lead to effective learning: a BEME systematic review. *Med Teach.*, **27**, 10–28.

4 Murphy, J.G., Cremonini, F., Kane, G.C. and Dunn, W. (2007) Is simulation based medicine training the future of clinical medicine? *Eur Rev Med Pharmacol Sci*, **11** (1), 1–8.

5 Ziv, A., Wolpe, P.R., Small, S.D. and Glick, S. (2003) Simulation-based medical education: an ethical imperative. *Acad Med*, **78** (8), 783–8.

6 Beauchamp, T.L. and Childress, J.F. (2009) *Principles of biomedical ethics*, 6th edn, Oxford University Press, New York.

7 Gutting G. Michel Foucault. In: Zalta EN, editor. *The Stanford encyclopedia of philosophy*. 2014. Available at: http://plato.stanford.edu/cgi-bin/encyclopedia/archinfo.cgi?entry=foucault.

8 Hodges, B.D., Martimianakis, M.A., McNaughton, N. and Whitehead, C. (2014) Medical education … meet Michel Foucault. *Med Educ*, **48** (6), 563–71.

9 Evans, L.V., Dodge, K.L., Shah, T.D. *et al.* (2010) Simulation training in central venous catheter insertion: improved performance in clinical practice. *Acad Med*, **85** (9), 1462–9.

10 McGaghie, W.C., Issenberg, S.B., Cohen, E.R. *et al.* (2011) Does simulation-based medical education with deliberate practice yield better results than traditional clinical education? A meta-analytic comparative review of the evidence. *Acad Med*, **86** (6), 706–11.

11 Zendejas, B., Brydges, R., Wang, A.T. and Cook, D.A. (2013) Patient outcomes in simulation-based medical education: a systematic review. *J Gen Intern Med*, **28** (8), 1078–89.

12 Finan, E., Bismilla, Z., Campbell, C. *et al.* (2012) Improved procedural performance following a simulation training session may not be transferable to the clinical environment. *J Perinatol*, **32** (7), 539–44.

13 Gillon, R. (1994) Medical ethics: four principles plus attention to scope. *BMJ*, **309** (6948), 184.

14 Tritrakarn, P., Berg, B.W., Kasuya, R.T. and Sakai, D.H. (2014) Medical school hotline: can we use simulation to teach medical ethics? *Hawaii J Med Public Health*, **73** (8), 262.

15 Nestel, D., Clark, S., Tabak, D. *et al.* (2010) Defining responsibilities of simulated patients in medical education. *Simul Healthc*, **5** (3), 161–8.

16 Bruppacher, H.R., Chen, R.P. and Lachapelle, K. (2011) First, do no harm: using simulated patient death to enhance learning. *Med Educ*, **45** (3), 317–18.

17 Bosk, C.L. (1981) *Forgive and remember: managing medical failure*, 2nd edn, University of Chicago Press, Chicago, IL.

18 Okuda, Y., Bryson, E.O., DeMaria, S. Jr., *et al.* (2009) The utility of simulation in medical education: what is the evidence? *Mt Sinai J Med.*, **76**, 330–43.

19 Zendejas, B., Wang, A.T., Brydges, R. *et al.* (2012) Cost: the missing outcome in simulation-based medical education research: a systematic review. *Surgery*, **153** (2), 160–76.

20 Martin, J. (2007) *Educational metamorphoses: philosophical reflections on identity and culture*, Rowman & Littlefield, New York.

21 Emmerich, N. (2013) *Medical ethics education: an interdisciplinary and social theoretical perspective*, Springer, London.

22 Emmerich, N. (2015) Bourdieu's collective enterprise of inculcation: the moral socialisation and ethical enculturation of medical students. *Brit J Sociol Educ*, **36** (7), 1054–72.

23 Levy, N. (2006) Foucault as virtue ethicist. *Foucault Stud.*, **1**, 20–31.

24 Schön, D.A. (1984) *The reflective practitioner: how professionals think in action*, Basic Books, New York.

25 Schön, A. (1990) *Educating the reflective practitioner: toward a new design for teaching and learning*, Jossey-Bass, San Francisco, CA.

26 Robinson R. Foucault, Michel : *ethics*. Internet encyclopedia of philosophy. 2011. Available at: http://www.iep.utm.edu/fouc-eth/

27 Ghaye, T. (2010) In what ways can reflective practices enhance human flourishing? *Reflect Pract*, **11** (1), 1–7.

28 Underman, K. (2015) Playing doctor: simulation in medical school as affective practice. *Soc Sci Med.*, **136–7**, 180–88.

CHAPTER 17

Teamwork and healthcare simulation

Jenny Weller & Ian Civil

KEY MESSAGES

- Failures in teamwork and communication between health-care providers account for a major burden of avoidable patient harm and treatment injuries.

- The curriculum for team training is well defined and based in theory and evidence, and simulation is an effective approach to delivering this curriculum.

- Teamwork training needs to involve teams who work together in order to overcome professional boundaries and needs to engage all members of the team in meaningful activities relevant to their professional roles.

- Development and delivery of multidisciplinary simulation-based team training requires a multidisciplinary faculty and organizational commitment to overcome the many barriers to implementation.

- Simulation-based team training should be embedded in healthcare institutions and become part of business as usual for quality improvement and patient safety.

Overview

Failures in teamwork and communication lead to tension, unhappy workplaces and error. There is good evidence that simulation training improves teamwork and communication and reduces the risk of peri-operative harm. Multidisciplinary simulation-based team training presents many challenges in terms of effective scenario design and the logistics of multidisciplinary attendance and 'buy-in'. Changes in the culture and expectations of both professional groups

and employers are necessary for effective simulation in teamwork and communication, but it is only with such change that the benefits can be realized.

Introduction

Modern healthcare is complex, multifaceted and often fragmented. Patients see many different health professionals over the course of a single illness. The extent to which their care is coordinated, and these health professionals communicate effectively and work as team, will to a very large extent influence the outcome for the patient [1]. Teamwork and communication between health professionals both have an important effect on patient outcomes through reducing errors, delays and disorganized patient care. Improving teamwork and communication could potentially bring about the most significant reductions in morbidity and mortality in modern healthcare.

However, health professionals have paid little attention to teamwork and communication between different health professional groups in traditional training programmes. Furthermore, it is common for training to occur in professional silos, from undergraduate programmes through to continuing professional development [2, 3]. The results are communication failures and sub-optimal teamwork in healthcare teams, particularly across professional boundaries. These failures have been documented by observations of healthcare teams in the clinical environment [4]. Adverse events are common, millions of hospitalized patients suffer

Healthcare Simulation Education: Evidence, Theory and Practice, First Edition.
Edited by Debra Nestel, Michelle Kelly, Brian Jolly and Marcus Watson.
© 2018 John Wiley & Sons Ltd. Published 2018 by John Wiley & Sons Ltd.

avoidable treatment injuries every year, and many of these are attributed to failures in communication [5–8]. Simulation-based training for multidisciplinary healthcare teams could be part of the solution to this problem.

Does Simulation-Based Team Training Work?

There are numerous reports of simulation-based team training across many disciplines [9–22]. These have demonstrated effectiveness in many different forms, including participant self-report, evidence of learning or improved performance in simulated cases, improved teamwork processes in the clinical environment, changes in attitudes towards safety, improved perceptions of clinical decision making and, in some cases, improved patient outcomes. While it is difficult in a single study to provide incontrovertible evidence of improved outcomes for patients, the combined evidence of the many published studies is overwhelming. In some regions, simulation has become embedded in institutional practice [23], but this is generally not the case, and the failure of institutions to act on this evidence is a cause for concern.

Key Considerations in Simulation-Based Team Training

Theoretical Framework for Effective Team Functioning

A theoretical framework for effective teamwork is a good starting point in developing simulation-based team training. Salas et al. [24] undertook an extensive review of the teamwork literature and developed a framework comprising five key dimensions and three underpinning mechanisms for effective teams. The key dimensions are team leadership, mutual performance monitoring, back-up behaviour, adaptability and team orientation. The underpinning mechanisms are mutual trust, closed-loop communication and shared mental models (Figure 17.1).

Each component can be considered in the context of healthcare team training. Members of the team must respect and trust each other in order to monitor each other's performance, speak up and give and receive advice or assistance on mistakes, lapses or task overload. Good communication is critical for sharing information and developing a shared mental model. Shared mental models of the situation, the plan for treatment, the

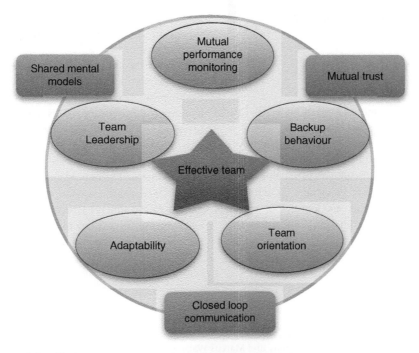

Figure 17.1 A framework for effective teams. Source: Adapted from Salas 2005 [24]

roles and tasks of other individuals in the team and future events enable team members to anticipate each other's needs, identify changes in the clinical situation and adapt accordingly. An effective leader coordinates tasks and treatment plans and is pivotal to the development of the team, and in establishing a positive team atmosphere. This framework provides a basis for a curriculum in simulation-based team training, and specific strategies and skills to enhance team performance. Alternative frameworks such as TeamSTEPPS have very similar sets of goals and frameworks supported via well-developed curricula [25].

A Curriculum for Training Healthcare Teams

A curriculum can be described in terms of knowledge, skills and attitudes, all relevant to the simulation-based training of healthcare teams.

Knowledge

The relevance of teamwork can be emphasized through the literature on error causation and the consequences of failures in teamwork. A theoretical framework for effective teamwork behaviors such as that proposed by Salas et al. [24] is essential to underpin behaviour change. An understanding of the issues of interprofessional collaboration and collective competence [2], the influence of hierarchies in healthcare teams and the construction of professional boundaries [26] underpins culture change.

Skills/behaviours

The skills and behaviours required for effective teamwork include managing the team (e.g. coordination, monitoring and supporting others); managing the task (e.g. role allocation, planning, prioritizing, identifying and utilizing resources); and developing a shared team mental model (information sharing on task and role). The communication skills underpinning effective teamwork include closed-loop communication, structured handover [27], call-out [28] and speaking up [29] (Table 17.1).

Measurement scales for teamwork behaviours often provide explicit descriptors of expected behaviours, which help both participants and instructors to recognize and develop these behaviours (Table 17.2).

Attitudes

Mutual trust and respect and a team orientation are key dimensions of effective teams. Clinicians need to be convinced of the relevance of learning about teamwork and communication in order to change, but important barriers exist. Bringing the different health professional groups together in simulation-based team training provides opportunities to learn about the roles

Table 17.1 Some useful communication behaviours.

Closed-loop communication	ISBAR (structured handover)	Call-out (SNAPPI) (call-out in a crisis)	Speaking up
Sender: clear, concise, directed instruction	Identify – who you are Situation – the main issue	**S**top – leader steps back and gets the attention of the team	**3-step CUS model** I am **C**oncerned
Receiver: read-back of instruction to ensure correct understanding	**B**ackground – the background history	**N**otify – inform the team of patient status	I am **U**ncomfortable This is a **S**afety issue
Sender: confirmation of instruction	**A**ssessment – what you think is going on	**A**ssessment – your interpretation of the situation	**4-step PACE model** Probe Alert
Receiver: acceptance of the task	**R**ecommendation – what you think needs to be done next	**P**lan – what you think needs to be done	Challenge Emergency
		Priorities – state the order for the plan	**Modified PACE model** Observation Suggestion
		Invite ideas – seek input from the team	Challenge Emergency

Table 17.2 Teamwork measurement tools.

OTAS – observational teamwork assessment for surgery [30]	Operating room teams: covers five behavior categories of three sub-teams (surgical, nursing, anaesthesia) over three phases of surgery
Teamwork Behavioral Rater [31]	Intensive care teams: covers 23 individual behavioural items that group into three main categories, rated over the entire encounter
Non-technical skills – ANTS [32]	Anaesthesia: covers four behaviour categories of performance, rated over the entire encounter

and capabilities of others and how they contribute to decision making and patient management. Hierarchical attitudes, where power differentials exist between team members, discourage open communication. The less powerful fear negative consequences, and the powerful fail to value the input of all team members [33]. Simulation-based team training brings different members of the team together on an equal footing. It can engage them in challenges designed to expose assumptions and behaviours that limit effective team function and result in sub-optimal care.

Simulation can be a powerful way of demonstrating what happens when teamwork and communication fail. Unlike other methods, such as a video demonstration, the experiential perspective provided through active participation in a simulated event can promote a deeper reflection on strategies to improve team effectiveness and patient care. Where participants display effective teamwork and communication in the simulation, the experience can be used to reflect on and promote behaviours that support good outcomes. Simulation provides many advantages over other training modalities, including the option of repeating an event to try out or practise new strategies. The opportunity for participants to meet and get to know each other during the training sessions should not be overlooked.

Practical Considerations

Effective multidisciplinary team training requires each member of the team to undertake activities similar to their normal tasks. In the operating theatre (OT) context, for example, this means that anaesthesiologists,

anaesthetic technicians, nurses and the surgical team must all have relevant clinical activities in which to engage during the simulation. An appropriate level of fidelity for each group is a prerequisite for this engagement. In this context, fidelity relates not only to the physical environment in which the simulation occurs, but also to the nature of the scenario that the simulation seeks to replicate. Mismatch in fidelity results in an 'observational' process where those with less to do simply watch the performance of those with more. It is apparent therefore that a multidisciplinary team is needed to provide input into scenario design to ensure appropriate balance.

Where suitable fidelity exists for the different professional groups, all participants can engage in realistic activities. Team members can then interact with each other in a similar way to their interactions in the clinical environment. Thus the realism is more about interactions between participants rather than interactions with the simulator.

For example, tasks that might form part of an OT scenario for which there should be similar levels of fidelity might include monitoring for the anaesthesiologist, control of surgical bleeding for the surgeon and maintaining sterility for the scrub nurse.

Multidisciplinary scenarios must be reasonably specific for the professional groups involved. For example, in the OT context, involving surgeons is probably more difficult than the other professional groups due to sub-specialism differences in surgical procedures. For example, a scenario about abdominal bleeding cannot be used for a neurosurgical team and, similarly, an extremity vascular scenario is of limited relevance to urologists. The temptation to go for a 'common denominator', such as skin incision, runs the risk of relative disengagement by the surgical participants unless some particular action is required of them. The less any individual group engages, the less teamwork can be simulated and thus the objective of the simulation may be defeated. Therefore, the challenge of creating realistic physical simulation models and believable scenarios is a particular challenge for simulations involving surgeons and necessitates a high level of surgical engagement in the simulation design team. Similar issues will apply in other healthcare contexts, particularly those involving invasive procedures or imaging techniques.

Briefing and Debriefing Multidisciplinary Teams

Much of the learning and application to practise from the simulation will occur in the debriefing. Factors to consider are seizing the opportunity to debrief interprofessional issues, and identifying and debriefing of issues of importance to all the different professional groups. Debriefing multidisciplinary teams exposes the particular challenges of communication and teamwork across professional boundaries, for example assumptions of shared understanding of the issues and plan for treatment; understanding others' roles and capabilities, and what they need to know to work most efficiently, as well as the difficulties in speaking up across hierarchies or professional boundaries. Opportunities for such discussions are so rarely otherwise available. Highlighting the opportunities for interprofessional learning when preparing participants for the simulation, and facilitating discussion around interprofessional issues as they arise in the debriefing, may help to address power gradients and interprofessional barriers in the clinical environment.

Again in the context of OT simulations, an anaesthesiologist debriefer may not be in the best position to notice and make explicit the issues that arose during the scenario for nursing staff. Ideally, a multidisciplinary instructor team should be involved in the debriefing. This requires planning and an agreed approach to the structure of the debriefing and the different roles that the debriefers will take. An option could be a non-clinical debriefer, not aligned with any particular professional group and trained in team-based debriefing.

Logistically this could mean that more faculty are required, and perhaps a rapid upskilling of some faculty to take on the role of debriefer. A structured format to debriefing can be of benefit to less experienced debriefers [34]. A useful structure is to begin with exploration of feelings or emotional reactions to the scenario, then clarification of the events during the scenario, followed by exploration of why certain things happened and how things could have been managed differently, and finally application of these simulated experiences and lessons learnt to clinical practice. Questioning techniques include questions of clarification, questions prompting self-reflection of what was done well and areas for improvement, and advocacy/inquiry [35], where the debriefer states their observation and potential concern and explores the reasoning or

rationale of the participants. With a multidisciplinary team of instructors, it is important that they share the same mental model – their plan for the debriefing, their various roles and who will do what (see Chapter 21).

Challenges in Teamwork Simulation

Appropriate Level of Fidelity of Simulation and Team Interactions

For teamwork simulation to be effective, every member of the team needs to be engaged and the interaction between them needs to have fidelity as well as their individual relationship with the simulation. Needless to say, the whole team needs to be represented in the scenario and the roles they are assigned should be as close as possible to the normal roles they fill in the clinical environment. In teamwork simulations as much effort needs to be put into the scenario as into the simulator.

Appropriate fidelity can be defined as that degree of realism that allows team members to suspend disbelief and engage in the scenario in a meaningful way. Chapter 4 provides a more detailed discussion on generating meaningful outcomes. Thus there is no precise degree of anatomical, physiological or facility fidelity that is required, but rather sufficient physical realism and scenario narrative that allow all participants to engage. Attention to all elements is critical during the briefing, conduct and debriefing to achieve effective teamwork simulation.

Logistical Challenges to Implementation

The need to engage all members of the multidisciplinary team presents both cost and logistic challenges. Many of these are similar to the barriers widely reported for undergraduate interprofessional education initiatives, for example timetabling; different weight for the assessment of the activity; and ensuring that learning objectives are equally relevant for all students [36].

In multidisciplinary healthcare teams, availability of the various team members as well as the culture of the health professional group to which they belong can be problematic. Issues including difference in funding, rosters and competing individual training needs will vary across professional groups. Some professional groups may struggle with the relevance of multidisciplinary team training to their own professional practice and require special efforts or incentives. This may affect the appropriate numbers of participants from each profession able to attend interprofessional education at external sites. While participation may be facilitated by using in situ simulation training, participants may be called away, and the simulation activity needs careful management so as not to detract from patient care [37].

Multidisciplinary simulation team training requires strategies that actively involve all groups. Again, this comes back to involving a multidisciplinary team at the outset, but also identifying champions in each clinical group and gaining organizational support.

Transfer from Simulation to Real World

One of the challenges of any simulation-based intervention is the degree to which learning and new insights transfer to the clinical workplace. In this regard, multidisciplinary teamwork simulation is no different from any other form of simulation. Whereas task-based simulation requires an individual's experience with the task to be recalled when in the real-life environment, team-based simulation aims for changes in the behaviour of whole teams. One factor affecting transfer may be the location in which the simulation is held. The mere fact that an individual may need to travel to a simulation environment other than their workplace, and potentially train with participants with whom they do not normally work, may affect learning transfer. The extent to which the learning and insights about teamwork and communication flourish and lead to changes in behaviour in the clinical workplace is likely to depend on the percentage of staff who attended the training and who can reinforce the lessons learnt.

Current Trends and Future Directions

In situ simulation has the advantage of providing immediate relevance to the workplace, but does place demands on the instructors to ensure that management of the scenario is safe and that fidelity is not compromised. Simulation centres have the benefit of a tightly managed environment and the opportunity to practise repeatedly in the same place, leading to a well-managed process, but this will inevitably result in geographical dissonance for the participants.

Perhaps the ideal compromise is a formal simulation environment close to or within the workplace (for example, one cubicle in the emergency department, or

one patient room in the intensive care unit, permanently used for simulation) [38]. In an environment where educators generally struggle to get employers (other than airlines and the military) to regard simulation as 'business as usual', this is a distant goal for many at the present time.

A single workshop is unlikely to have a prolonged effect. To promote permanent change in culture and retention of knowledge, skills and behaviours, the intervention needs to be recurrent and embedded, to become part of normal business. The 'stickiness' of the intervention will depend on the ability to engage the majority of members of departments, the clear relevance and evidence of the benefits of the training, and regular reinforcement through repeated training and organizational support.

Some areas of clinical practice have embraced multidisciplinary simulation-based team training to a far greater extent than others, in particular OT teams, obstetrics, emergency medicine and intensive care. These are typically the areas of acute care practice, where outcomes are closely linked to immediate management and where senior clinicians are involved. Extending teamwork training to ward staff, including junior doctors involved in acute response to the deteriorating patient, and further to more routine or chronic care, are areas for future exploration.

A key dimension of teamwork is team orientation – an attitude that recognizes the value of teamwork, information sharing and team decision making in optimizing patient care and safety. Optimal multidisciplinary teamwork simulation could potentially produce such a change in the culture of the participants through carefully crafted scenarios and debriefings designed to expose the inefficiencies and potential hazards of entrenched hierarchies and individualistic attitudes. Simulation can also be used to demonstrate the advantages of flattened hierarchies, environments that encourage speaking up, and the implementation of safety interventions designed to enhance information sharing between health practitioners, such as the WHO Surgical Safety Checklist [38].

Conclusion

Bringing health professionals together in multidisciplinary simulation-based team training enables teams that work together to learn how to communicate more effectively with each other and work collaboratively in patient-centred healthcare teams. While challenges exist in incorporating simulation-based team training into healthcare organizations as part of 'business as usual', the potential for improvements in patient safety and reductions in avoidable harm could be significant.

References

1 Mazzocco, K., Petitti, D.B., Fong, K.T. *et al.* (2009) Surgical team behaviors and patient outcomes. *Am J Surg.*, **197**, 678–85.

2 Hodges, B. and Lingard, L. (2012) *The question of competence: reconsidering medical education in the twenty first century*, Cornell University Press, Ithaca, NY.

3 Baker, D.P., Salas, E., King, H. *et al.* (2005) The role of teamwork in the professional education of physicians: current status and assessment recommendations. *Jt Comm J Qual Patient Saf.*, **31**, 185–202.

4 Lingard, L., Espin, S., Whyte, S. *et al.* (2004) Communication failures in the operating room: an observational classification of recurrent types and effects. *Qual Saf Health Care.*, **13**, 330–34.

5 Jha, A.K., Larizgoitia, I., Audera-Lopez, C. *et al.* (2013) The global burden of unsafe medical care: analytic modelling of observational studies. *BMJ Qual Saf.*, **22**, 809–15.

6 Davis, P., Lay-Yee, R., Briant, R. *et al.* (2002) Adverse events in New Zealand public hospitals I: occurrence and impact. *N Z Med J.*, **115**, 271–7.

7 Leape, L., Brennan, T., Laird, N. *et al.* (1991) The nature of adverse events in hospitalized patients: the results of the Harvard Medical Practice Study II. *N Engl J Med.*, **324**, 377–84.

8 Vincent, C., Neale, G. and Woloshynowych, M. (2001) Adverse events in British hospitals: preliminary retrospective record review. *BMJ.*, **322**, 517–19.

9 Tan, S.B., Pena, G., Altree, M. and Maddern, G.J. (2014) Multidisciplinary team simulation for the operating theatre: a review of the literature. *ANZ J Surg.*, **84**, 515–22.

10 Merién, A.E.R., van de Ven, J., Mol, B.W. *et al.* (2010) Multidisciplinary team training in a simulation setting for acute obstetric emergencies: a systematic review. *Obstet Gynecol.*, **115**, 1021–31.

11 Undre, S., Koutantji, M., Sevdalis, N. *et al.* (2007) Multidisciplinary crisis simulations: the way forward for training surgical teams. *World J Surg.*, **31**, 1843–53.

12 Falcone, R.A. Jr., Daugherty, M., Schweer, L. *et al.* (2008) Multidisciplinary pediatric trauma team training using high-fidelity trauma simulation. *J Pediatr Surg.*, **43**, 1065–71.

13 Steinemann, S., Berg, B., Skinner, A. *et al.* (2011) In situ, multidisciplinary, simulation-based teamwork training improves early trauma care. *J Surg Educ.*, **68**, 472–7.

14 Allan, C.K., Thiagarajan, R.R., Beke, D. *et al.* (2010) Simulation-based training delivered directly to the pediatric cardiac intensive care unit engenders preparedness, comfort, and decreased anxiety among multidisciplinary resuscitation teams. *J Thorac Cardiovasc Surg.*, **140**, 646–52.

15 Nishisaki, A., Nguyen, J., Colborn, S. *et al.* (2011) Evaluation of multidisciplinary simulation training on clinical performance and team behavior during tracheal intubation procedures in a pediatric intensive care unit. *Pediatr Crit Care Med.*, **12**, 406–14.

16 Robertson, B., Kaplan, B., Atallah, H. *et al.* (2010) The use of simulation and a modified teamstepps curriculum for medical and nursing student team training. *Simul Healthc.*, **5**, 332–7.

17 Weaver, S.J., Dy, S.M. and Rosen, M.A. (2014) Team-training in healthcare: a narrative synthesis of the literature. *BMJ Qual Saf.*, **23**, 359–72.

18 Riley, W., Davis, S., Miller, K. *et al.* (2011) Didactic and simulation nontechnical skills team training to improve perinatal patient outcomes in a community hospital. *Jt Comm J Qual Patient Saf.*, **37**, 357–64.

19 Maxson, P.M., Dozois, E.J., Holubar, S.D. *et al.* (2011) Enhancing nurse and physician collaboration in clinical decision making through high-fidelity interdisciplinary simulation training. *Mayo Clin Proc.*, **86**, 31–6.

20 Cumin, D., Boyd, M.J., Webster, C.S. and Weller, J.M. (2013) A systematic review of simulation for multidisciplinary team training in operating rooms. *Simul Healthc.*, **8**, 171–9.

21 Frengley, R.W., Weller, J., Torrie, J. *et al.* (2011) The effect of a simulation-based training intervention on the performance of established critical care unit teams. *Crit Care Med.*, **39**, 2605–11.

22 Weller, J., Cumin, D., Torrie, J. *et al.* (2015) Multidisciplinary operating room simulation-based team training to reduce treatment errors: a feasibility study in New Zealand hospitals. *N Z Med J.*, **128**, 1418.

23 Arriaga, A.F., Gawande, A.A., Raemer, D.B. *et al.* (2014) Pilot testing of a model for insurer-driven, large-scale multicenter simulation training for operating room teams. *Ann Surg.*, **259**, 403–10.

24 Salas, E., Sims, D.E. and Burke, C.S. (2005) Is there a 'Big Five' in teamwork? *Small Group Res.*, **36**, 555–99.

25 AHRQ. TeamSTEPPS: strategies and tools to enhance performance and patient safety [cited 1 September 2016]. Available at: http://www.ahrq.gov/professionals/education/curriculum-tools/teamstepps/index.html

26 Weller, J. (2012) Shedding new light on tribalism in health care. *Med Educ.*, **46**, 134–6.

27 Marshall, S., Harrison, J. and Flanagan, B. (2009) The teaching of a structured tool improves the clarity and content

of interprofessional clinical communication. *Qual Saf Health Care.*, **18**, 137–40.

28 Weller, J.M., Torrie, J., Boyd, M. *et al.* (2014) Improving team information sharing with a structured call-out in anaesthetic emergencies: a randomized controlled trial. *Br J Anaesth.*, **112**, 1042–9.

29 Rutherford, J.S., Flin, R. and Mitchell, L. (2012) Teamwork, communication, and anaesthetic assistance in Scotland. *Br J Anaesth.*, **109**, 21–6.

30 Passauer-Baierl, S., Hull, L., Miskovic, D. *et al.* (2014) Re-validating the Observational Teamwork Assessment for Surgery tool (OTAS-D): cultural adaptation, refinement, and psychometric evaluation. *World J Surg.*, **38**, 305–13.

31 Weller, J., Frengley, R., Torrie, J. *et al.* (2011) Evaluation of an instrument to measure teamwork in multidisciplinary critical care teams. *BMJ Qual Saf.*, **20**, 216–22.

32 Fletcher, G., Flin, R., McGeorge, P. *et al.* (2003) Anaesthetists' non-technical skills (ANTS): evaluation of a behavioural marker system. *Brit J Anaesthes.*, **90**, 580–8.

33 Lichtenstein, R., Alexander, J.A., McCarthy, J.F. and Wells, R. (2004) Status differences in cross-functional teams: effects on individual member participation, job satisfaction, and intent to quit. *J Health Soc Behav.*, **45**, 322–35.

34 Eppich, W. and Cheng, A. (2015) Promoting excellence and reflective learning in simulation (PEARLS): development and rationale for a blended approach to health care simulation debriefing. *Simul Healthc.*, **10**, 106–15.

35 Rudolph, J.W., Simon, R., Dufresne, R.L. and Raemer, D.B. (2006) There's no such thing as 'nonjudgmental' debriefing: a theory and method for debriefing with good judgment. *Simul Healthc.*, **1**, 49–55.

36 Gilbert, J.H.V. (2005) Interprofessional learning and higher education structural barriers. *J Interprof Care*, **19** (suppl 1), 87–106.

37 Gaba, D.M. (2004) The future vision of simulation in health care. *Qual Saf Health Care.*, **13**, i2–i10. doi: 10.1136/qshc.2004.009878

38 Haynes, A., Weiser, T., Berry, W. *et al.* (2009) A surgical safety checklist to reduce morbidity and mortality in a global population. *N Engl J Med.*, **360**, 491–9.

CHAPTER 18

Designing simulation-based learning activities: A systematic approach

Debra Nestel & Suzanne Gough

KEY MESSAGES

- The literature reports many approaches to designing simulations and simulation frameworks.
- Systematic approaches can assist the quality of the educational experience.
- Irrespective of simulation modality, professional discipline and setting, there are commonalities in simulation-based education.
- Phases of simulation include preparing, briefing, simulation activity, debriefing/feedback, reflecting and evaluating.

Overview

In this chapter we provide an overview of simulation practices relevant for any immersive simulation experience. We start by describing a simulation framework used in a national training programme in Australia (NHET-Sim): preparing, briefing, simulation activity, debriefing/feedback, reflecting and evaluating. We illustrate the simulation phases using a hybrid simulation for learner surgeons in a formative assessment. We acknowledge that there are many approaches and offer this as one that has widespread application.

Introduction

The literature offers several valuable approaches to designing simulation-based learning activities. For example, Jeffries published a simulation framework for application in nursing education [1]. Dieckmann based his framework on interprofessional mannequin-based simulations [2], while Gough describes a framework for simulation derived from her studies in cardiorespiratory physiotherapy education [3]. Although from different professional practices and based on different simulation modalities, these frameworks have commonalities that reflect effective educational design. Systematic approaches to simulation design can strengthen practice and promote learning [4, 5]. Chapter 2 acknowledges theories that inform healthcare simulation education, including deliberate practice, which offers further guidance to simulation practice.

Simulation practices are also informed by standards offered by professional associations (see the additional resources at the end of this chapter). These standards have relevance at different levels of application: centre, programme, scenarios, facilitators and so on. Our focus in this chapter is consideration of simulation design at the level of the individual simulation event.

We use a systematic approach offered by a national simulation educator programme in Australia [6]. The NHET-Sim programme was designed for individuals working with any simulation modality, in any setting and across professions. The systematic approach focuses on the design of simulation events rather than a whole curriculum, but can be scaled to accommodate the system in which the simulation event is to be located; that is, the broader workplace and curriculum activities of the learners. The phases enable practitioners to share a common language for designing and communicating about simulation-based education (SBE). We illustrate this systematic approach with a simulation designed to support trainee surgeons in managing effective communication with a patient undergoing removal of a mole (Box 18.1).

Healthcare Simulation Education: Evidence, Theory and Practice, First Edition.
Edited by Debra Nestel, Michelle Kelly, Brian Jolly and Marcus Watson.
© 2018 John Wiley & Sons Ltd. Published 2018 by John Wiley & Sons Ltd.

Box 18.1 An example of a hybrid simulation using the NHET-Sim programme's six phases.

Preparing

Topic
Removal of a mole

Summary
Mr Brian Remington has come for removal of a mole on his upper arm. He is cooperative, although anxious because his sister died from malignant melanoma and he is concerned this may be a melanoma. The surgeon will explain the procedure, inject anaesthesia and close the wound.

Learning objectives
Trainee surgeon demonstrates competence in:
- Identifying the correct patient
- Explaining the procedure
- Identifying and acknowledging the patient's concerns
- Making empathic statements
- Communicating with the patient while operating
- Communicating with the nurse
- Checking the patient knows the next steps

Requirements

Simulated patient	Dissection and
Nurse to assist	suturing instruments
Simulated patient's	Specimen container
notes/patient chart	for pathology
Barrier sheet	Trolley
Fenestrated drape	Suturing pack
Mole model/skin pad	Sutures
Velcrose holder	Sterile gloves
Procedure/operating	Local anaesthetic –
room	Lignocaine 1% plain
Chairs	Syringes (5 ml and
Procedure couch	10 ml)
Mole skin pad with	Needles (green and
perspex holder	blue)
Fenestrated	Sharps container
adhesive disposal drape	Bin

Task for trainee surgeon
Mr Brian Remington has come to the day surgery clinic for removal of a mole on his arm. You are required to manage the consultation and remove the mole.

Information for the simulated patient (SP)
You are Mr. Brian Remington, aged 56, and you have come for removal of a mole on your upper right arm. You are cooperative, although anxious because your sister died from malignant melanoma four years ago. The surgeon will explain the procedure, inject anaesthesia and close the wound. The learning objectives are as listed earlier.

Behaviour
You are cooperative and communicative, but you have an underlying worry about cancer.

SP questions and prompts
Answer the trainee's questions honestly, but do not elaborate information unless the trainee facilitates this by pausing and staying with your answers. While the trainee is removing the mole, mention that your sister died of skin cancer. If the trainee acknowledges what you have said, then go on to ask if your mole could be malignant. Our experience is that often the trainees do not hear or acknowledge your comment while they are operating.

If information is not presented about the removal of the stitches, ask about what happens next towards the end of the interaction. 'Do these stitches just dissolve?' 'How do I get them removed?' Other questions to ask across the interaction, depending on the flow of communication, include: 'What exactly is a mole?' 'Why do people get them?' 'Will it come back?' 'Will I get others and what should I do about it?' At some point touch the drape while the trainee is watching unless they have already asked you not to do so.

In addition to considering the communication issues that occur during the procedure, there are a number of other points in playing this role. The trainee needs to inject local anaesthesia prior to the mole being removed. The injection will sting, so grimace. Sometimes trainees ask you to look away, but you need to watch so that you can respond at the precise moment. The trainee will wait a short time (a couple of minutes) and then is likely to test the site for numbness by poking around it with a blunt instrument. If asked if you can feel anything, say 'no'.

The trainee will use a cutting instrument to remove the mole and then stitch it closed.

Do not engage the nurse in conversation unless the trainee promotes discussion.

You are concerned that you may have cancer and also about the scarring on your arm ('I remember my sister had a great hole on her shoulder. It was really disfiguring.')

History of present illness
You first noticed the mole six months ago. Two weeks ago, you visited your general practitioner (GP). Your GP assessed the mole and believes that it is benign, but has referred you to the hospital for removal of the mole. The mole has not

grown in size since you first noticed. You are concerned that it might be cancer because of your sister's history.

Past medical history

Nothing significant.

Social history

You are a landscape gardener – you will need to get back to work. Your parents are alive and have no health problems. You sister had a mole on her left shoulder for several years, but it changed about two years before she died. 'She had it removed a couple of years before she died, but obviously it had already become malignant. It was terrible. Still is difficult. Her kids are managing though. Amazing what kids can handle.'

Family history

You are married to Susan and a father of two boys, Joseph (aged 14) and Lewis (aged 16).

Considerations in playing this role

You will have a suture pad velcroed around your right upper arm (wear a short-sleeved top that is not bulky) and the pad will have a surgical drape covering it to create the impression that the mole is on your arm. The pad has a hard perspex backing to protect your arm and can get uncomfortable, so we will remove it whenever possible.

Briefing

The facilitator briefs the trainees. In addition to the usual actions described in the text, including sharing the learning objectives, the facilitator seeks the following information:

- Have you done this procedure before? In the skills lab? With real patients? How did it go?
- How are you feeling? How confident are you? How competent do you think you are at this? What are the most likely challenges you will face? How do you think you will deal with them? Have you conducted any similar procedures? Are there similar skills needed for this procedure? How easy/hard will it be to use them here?
- What did you do well the last time you did this procedure?
- Did you have any particular difficulties? If so, what were they?
- What are you most hoping to learn?
- What would you like us to observe?
- From the patient's and nurse's perspective, is there anything you would like feedback on?

The facilitator allocates tasks for the observers (other trainees).

Simulating

The facilitator observes.

Debriefing/feedback

The focus of the debriefing/feedback relates to exploring how the trainee felt during the procedure, what went well and identifying what did not go so well/as planned. The facilitator should invite the SP and observer trainees to offer their perspective and draw on information from any observational rating tool (Table 18.1). This is crucial for developing the trainees' insight. Self-regulated learning goals may be discussed and, where a trainee has indicated specific points to be observed, feedback should be provided, drawing again on the SP and observers. Finally, how will the trainees make use of the experience? It is important to make a summary of what has been discussed and refer trainees to review any digital resources provided (e.g. a DVD of the simulation). Alternatively, other debriefing tools can be used to structure the discussion [7,8].

Reflecting

During the debriefing/feedback, ask learners to think about how they may apply this learning experience to their practice. What is similar? What is different? What conditions will align? What will be different? How will they check on whether they are progressing? What further practice do they require?

Evaluating

Faculty including SPs and learners will be asked to consider the extent to which the simulation event enabled them to meet the learning objectives. For the faculty, was there enough time?

Source: Adapted from a scenario developed for the ICARUS research project, Imperial College, London. Authored by D. Nestel, R. Kneebone and R. Aggarwal.

Figure 18.1 illustrates the phases and their cyclical relationship. The figure appears in its most basic form and can be adjusted to accommodate contextual variations. The *preparing* phase refers to all the activities that take place before the simulation event starts, such as identifying learners' needs; setting learning objectives; designing the scenario, sourcing simulators, medical equipment, props and so on; booking rooms; recruiting and identifying faculty, confederates and simulated patients (SPs); scheduling the learners; catering and so on. The range of tasks will depend on the local simulation facility and practices.

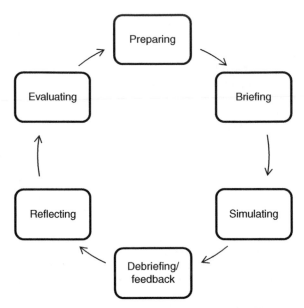

Figure 18.1 Phases in simulation design. Source: Adapted from the NHET-Sim Programme.

In our example, the activities associated with *preparing* will include identifying competencies required for learners, their prior experiences, anticipated challenges for learner(s) and so on. Given that the scenario (in Box 18.1) involves communication, an SP-based scenario is most likely to be appropriate, and because the task involves a procedural skill that can be easily simulated with a task trainer, a hybrid simulation will be suitable. The scenario will need to be developed to offer a level of sufficient challenge to learners. When working with groups of learners, this is complex because of variation in their levels of experience with the procedure. Approaches to scenario design vary and when SP based usually include an SP role in which the character and personal history of the SP are set out, as well as clinical features relevant to this particular scenario [3, 6]. To ensure that a patient voice is represented, seeking advice from lay people and SPs is important to ensure authenticity and feasibility. The SP will need to be trained to play the role, including in the extent to which standardization is important. As this scenario is being used in a formative assessment, a tight 'bandwidth' of performance will be less important than if the scenario was a summative assessment. The scenario may trigger an emotional response for the SP that could make their

performance unsettling for them, so they will need to be asked whether they think they will be able to manage. Approaches to training SPs are beyond the scope of this chapter, but refer to the additional resources.

The simulated setting in which the simulation takes place will need to be created, and consumables and other medical equipment checked for availability and functionality. It is important to do a 'run-through' of the whole procedure to ensure that the timings are appropriate for the task. Positioning of the SP and equipment within the setting will also need to be tested to ensure that observers have audiovisual access. The debriefing will be facilitator led and observers will use the rating form in Table 18.1. In this scenario, the SP will provide verbal feedback on the learner's performances with respect to the learning objectives. The facilitator will assist them in sharing this information using a protocol.

The *briefing* phase is given relatively little attention in the literature, but is really important in setting up valuable learning experiences [3]. To other faculty and SPs, the briefing will include the learning objectives, the learners' characteristics, logistics such as time frames, starting, pausing and ending the simulation activity, simulator programming, technical support, communication with the control room, audiovisual capacity, debriefing and feedback processes, reflective exercises and evaluation forms. Additionally, during the briefing it can be important to explore faculty's prior experiences of the scenario and their feelings about it. An opportunity for final questions can ensure smooth functioning. Sometimes SPs are briefed separately to learners for their first encounter within the simulation. Briefing learners will include most of these elements and may also include inviting learners to set their own goals relative to those prescribed and their experiences [9]. We provide an example in Box 18.1.

Orientation of learners to the simulation is important. This will include explicit discussion on what is similar and what is different to reality. This is linked to what is called a *fiction contract*.

Some learners find simulation stressful and it may be important to normalize the experience during the briefing. This involves acknowledgement that learners often find simulations stressful. Creating a safe learning environment involves several strategies and learner-centred attitudes from faculty. This can be achieved through several strategies, including clear explanation of the

Table 18.1 Observational rating form.

Patient-focused communication skills for procedural skills		Not done	Done incorrectly	Done correctly
	Opening			
1	Greeting	0	0	1
2	Introduction	0	0	1
	full name			
	– role	0	0	1
3	States purpose of procedure	0	0	1
4	Assesses patient's understanding of procedure	0	0	1
5	Establishes consent/agreement to proceed	0	0	1
6	Asks if patient has any questions	0	0	1
7	Asks if patient has any worries or concerns	0	0	1
	During procedure			
8	Explains procedure appropriately	0	0	1
	Closure			
9	States what has been done	0	0	1
10	States what will happen next	0	0	1
11	Checks patient's comfort	0	0	1
12	Checks patient's understanding	0	0	1
13	Asks if patient has any questions	0	0	1
14	Thanks the patient	0	0	1

Appropriate use of non-verbal communication (e.g. eye contact, body language, touch, facial expressions)

Not at all		Sometimes		Consistently
1	2	3	4	5

Responds to patient's verbal cues (e.g. questions, requests for explanations, worries)

Not at all		Sometimes		Consistently
1	2	3	4	5

Responds to patient's non-verbal cues (e.g. facial expression of discomfort)

Not at all		Sometimes		Consistently
1	2	3	4	5

Appropriate use of silence

Never		Sometimes		Always
1	2	3	4	5

Uses unexplained jargon

Throughout		Sometimes		Not at all
1	2	3	4	5

Interrupts patient appropriately

Never		Sometimes		Always
1	2	3	4	5

Makes empathic statements

Never		Occasionally		Throughout
1	2	3	4	5

Shows warmth

Never		Occasionally		Throughout
1	2	3	4	5

Perception of clinician's anxiety

Very anxious		Moderately anxious		Not at all anxious
1	2	3	4	5

Overall rating of patient-centred communication skills

Very poor		Satisfactory		Excellent
1	2	3	4	5

Comments:

simulation phases and their responsibilities in each, clarity over who is observing, what will happen with audio-visual recordings, confidentiality among those involved, seeking their buy-in with respect to doing their best, the orientation or familiarization of the simulators and setting.

During the *simulation activity* the learner(s) participate in the simulation. It is important to indicate a clear start to the simulation and observe for the physical and psychological safety of those within the simulation [5]. Minimal talking is often desirable to facilitate acute observation. Encouraging observers to make notes to enable specific feedback during debriefing can be valuable (see Box 18.1). If there is a pause and discuss option, then enact it as planned. Respond to cues for finishing the scenario. Depending on the simulation modalities, during the simulation activity cues may need to be pre-programmed onto the simulators (e.g. mannequin) and/or given to confederates, SPs and learners [4, 5]. Facilitators often develop their own approach to notation (electronic or hand written) and should be ready to commence as the simulation starts.

Once the simulation is over, observations of participants and observers can be really important in helping the facilitator to frame the opening debriefing statements. During this transition period there can be a lot of emotion expressed that is relevant to the debriefing and feedback. Encouraging participants to regroup and spend a few minutes thinking about what has just happened can be useful, including asking them to think about what worked well and what could have been improved. If observer tools are being used, then this is a good time to complete them (an example is provided in Box 18.1).

On ending the scenario, participants move to the debriefing room. It is helpful to organize the physical space, paying attention to seating arrangements, whiteboard and/or TV screen if video-assisted debriefing is used. As facilitator, it is helpful to have the learning objectives in your notes in order to stay focused. It is easy to be completely sidetracked by participants' responses. Remember to turn off recording devices. Follow the processes outlined in the briefing, although flexibility is also important to ensure learner-centredness. Invite observers, confederates and SPs to participate. Use opportunities, especially for communication-based scenarios, to rehearse micro elements of the scenario. This can be a valuable way of getting observers involved.

The *debriefing and feedback* phase complements the briefing, almost as bookends to the simulation activity. See Chapter 21 for further information. This phase is often reported to be the most important part of SBE that leads to learning [10–12]. Facilitators explore participants' feelings, address goals and learning objectives, seek other perspectives, summarize, affirm positive behaviours, explore unplanned issues and seek to establish new goals [13]. One goal of the debriefing is to promote reflection. However, we include this as a separate phase to highlight the importance of the locus of control for learning residing with the learner once they have left the simulation event.

Evidence of the effectiveness of debriefing has been reported [10, 11, 13–17]. Debriefing formats vary and debriefing is usually undertaken immediately after the simulation event (warm) or delayed (cold) [18]. Formats can be relatively unstructured to highly structured. Examples of debriefing tools, including the *diamond debrief* [7] and others, are provided in the London Handbook of Debriefing [18]. Similarly, debriefer rating tools such as the Objective Structured Assessment of Debriefing [6, 7, 18] and The Debriefing Assessment for Simulation in Healthcare [19] have been developed to provide evidence-based guidelines for conducting debriefings in simulated and real clinical settings. Guidelines for video-assisted debriefing have been published [20–23], but their optimal use remains unclear.

For the *reflecting* phase, learners (usually individually) are encouraged to make sense of the simulation in the light of their own experiences and those they plan. Similarly, faculty and SPs are encouraged to reflect on all facets of their contributions too. Reflecting is usually an individual activity; while debriefing is often collective and connected to the simulation activity, reflecting has a wider reach. During briefing, learners can be informed of reflecting activities and reinforced after the debriefing. Of course, there is overlap between these phases and reflecting can occur before the debriefing. There are several approaches to reflecting that have been adopted in SBE [24–26].

Learners can be directed to evidence their reflective practice following simulations by uploading and tagging digital learning resources (audio, photographs, video and podcasts etc.), within an e-portfolio [3] or blogs, social networking sites and wikis. Permissions need to be considered with respect to use and storage of these images. A case study using video reflexivity following simulation is provided in Chapter 23.

Evaluating refers to the success and limitations of the session in meeting its goals, rather than assessment of the individual. This phase benefits from the involvement of all stakeholders, although in practice it is often only learners, faculty, confederates and SPs who participate. It is well recognized in the literature and evident in simulation frameworks that evaluation is a crucial element of driving improvements in education, healthcare practice and ultimately patient care [1, 3].

While it is essential to consider the degree to which the SBE intervention has supported learning, meaningful evaluations require more sophisticated methods. Complex learning interventions require equally complex evaluations, using qualitative and quantitative methods to draw on multiple sources and triangulating data alongside exploring multiple levels of impact.

Conclusion

This chapter has introduced systematic simulation practices relevant for any immersive simulation experience. We acknowledge the restriction of the depth and detail permitted within the chapter, in relation to the phases and theoretical approaches underpinning the design, development and evaluation of SBE. However, reference has been made to other chapters within this book where more specific detail and examples can be located. This chapter has explored a systematic approach offered by an Australian national simulation educator programme and provided exemplar resources in Box 18.1.

References

1 Jeffries, P. (2005) A framework for designing, implementing, and evaluating simulations. *Nurs Educ Perspect*, **26** (2), 97–104.

2 Dieckmann, P. (ed.) (2009) *Using simulations for education, training and research*, Pabst, Lengerich.

3 Gough, S. (2016) *The use of simulation-based education in cardio-respiratory physiotherapy*, Unpublished doctoral thesis, Manchester Metropolitan University, Manchester.

4 Jeffries, P. (ed.) (2012) *Simulation in nursing education: from conceptualization to evaluation*, 2nd edn, National League for Nursing, New York.

5 Fenwick, T. and Dahlgren, M.A. (2015) Towards socio-material approaches in simulation-based education: lessons from complexity theory. *Med Educ*, **49** (4), 359–67.

6 Arora, S., Ahmed, M., Paige, J. et al. (2012) Objective structured assessment of debriefing (osad): bringing science to the art of debriefing in surgery. *Ann Surg*, **256** (6), 982–8.

7 Runnacles, J., Thomas, L., Sevdalis, N. et al. (2014) Development of a tool to improve performance debriefing and learning: the paediatric objective structured assessment of debriefing (OSAD) tool. *Postgrad Med J*, **90** (1069), 613–21.

8 NHET-Sim Monash Team. The National Health Education and Training – Simulation (NHET-Sim) programme. [cited 29 October 2012]. Available at: http://www.nhet-sim.edu.au/nhet-sim-program-3/overview/

9 Kneebone, R. and Nestel, D. (2005) Learning clinical skills: the place of simulation and feedback. *Clin Teach*, **2** (2), 86–90.

10 Issenberg, S.B., McGaghie, W.C., Petrusa, E.R. et al. (2005) Features and uses of high-fidelity medical simulations that lead to effective learning: a BEME systematic review. *Med Teach*, **27** (1), 10–28.

11 Motola, I., Devine, L.A., Chung, H.S. et al. (2013) Simulation in healthcare education: a best evidence practical guide. AMEE guide no. 82. *Med Teach*, **35** (1), e1511–e1530.

12 Shinnick, M.A., Woo, M., Horwich, T.B. and Steadman, R. (2011) Debriefing: the most important component in simulation? *Clin Simul Nurs.*, **7** (3) e105–e111.

13 Decker, S., Fey, M., Sideras, S. et al. (2013) Standards of best practice: simulation standard VI: the debriefing process. *Clin Simul Nurs*, **9** (6), S26–S29.

14 Fanning, R.M. and Gaba, D.M. (2007) The role of debriefing in simulation-based learning. *Simul Healthc*, **2** (2), 115–25.

15 Cheng, A., Eppich, W., Grant, V. et al. (2014) Debriefing for technology-enhanced simulation: a systematic review and meta-analysis. *Med Educ*, **48** (7), 657–66.

16 Rudolph, J.W., Simon, R., Dufresne, R.L. and Raemer, D.B. (2006) There's no such thing as 'nonjudgmental' debriefing: a theory and method for debriefing with good judgment. *Simul Healthc*, **1** (1), 49–55.

17 Benbow, E.W., Harrison, I., Dornan, T.L. and O'Neill, P.A. (1998) Pathology and the OSCE: insights from pilot study. *J Pathol*, **184** (1), 110–14.

18 Imperial College London (2012) *The London handbook for debriefing: enhancing performance debriefing in clinical and simulated settings*, London Deanery, London.

19 Centre for Medical Simulation. Debriefing assessment for simulation in healthcare (DASH©) [cited 1 May 2013]. Available at: http://www.harvardmedsim.org/debriefing-assesment-simulation-healthcare.php

20 Krogh, K., Bearman, M. and Nestel, D. (2015) Expert practice of video-assisted debriefing. *Clin Simul Nurs.*, **11** (3) e180–e187.

21 Grant, D.J. and Marriage, S.C. (2012) Training using medical simulation. *Arch Dis Child*, **97** (3), 255–9.

22 Grant, J.S., Moss, J., Epps, C. and Watts, P. (2010) Using video-facilitated feedback to improve student performance following high-fidelity simulation. *Clin Simul Nurs*, **6** (5), e177–e184.

23 Levett-Jones, T. and Lapkin, S. (2013) A systematic review of the effectiveness of simulation debriefing in health professional education. *Nurs Educ Today*, **34** (6), e58–e63.

24 Husebo, S., O'Regan, S. and Nestel, D. (2015) Reflective practice and its role in simulation. *Clin Simul Nurs.*, **11** (8) e368–e375.

25 Schön, D. (1987) *Educating the Reflective Practitioner*, Jossey-Bass, San Francisco, CA.

26 Kolb, D. and Fry, R. (1975) Toward an applied theory of experiential learning, in *Theories of group process* (ed. C. Cooper), John Wiley, Chichester.

Additional Resources

1 http://www.inacsl.org/i4a/pages/index.cfm?pageid=3407: A link to the standards associated with simulation as proposed by the International Nursing Association for Clinical Simulation and Learning.

2 http://www.sih.org: The Society for Simulation in Healthcare, for core standards and teaching and education standards.

3 www.spn.org: The Simulated Patient Network, a website that provides information for training simulated patients to participate in simulations.

CHAPTER 19

Facilitating healthcare simulations

Michelle Kelly & Stephen Guinea

KEY MESSAGES

- Flexibility is a key consideration when determining the level of facilitation during simulations.

- Don't assume 'participant/s should know what to do or how to respond'.

- Multiple factors may have impacts on the level of support required when facilitating simulations.

- Nuanced facilitation is ideal – knowing when to come in and out of the action.

- Facilitation should articulate with other components of simulations, particularly the debriefing processes and ongoing reflections.

Overview

Facilitating healthcare simulations can be considered from at least two perspectives: the role and attributes of the facilitator and the process of facilitation. Depending on participants' learning needs and the simulation objectives, the degree of facilitation will vary. However, there is general agreement that a level of guidance in the form of facilitation is required to help participants progress through a planned simulation experience, and to ensure that the learning objectives are achieved.

Within this chapter, we discuss the role of the facilitator and ways of facilitating simulations in the context of undergraduate nursing students within a Bachelor degree program. The practices and experiences of both authors, which frame these discussions, can be applied to other health disciplines or in situations where participants are in the early stages of embarking on a new clinical specialism or have rejoined the workforce after

an absence. To avoid overlap, references are provided to other chapters within this book that offer discussion about related topics.

Introduction

In essence, the core aim of healthcare simulations is to facilitate learning of, and about, practice [1]. Hence the role of the simulation facilitator is complex and requires a level of expertise in educational techniques and insight about the context of the scenario at hand, to assist participants in linking the experience of simulation to practice [2, 3].

Facilitation, as used within the context of this chapter, refers to collaborative, participative processes of learning characterized by guidance, support and engagement. Interactions between the facilitator and participants are about the co-production of knowledge – exploring the situation being simulated by drawing out participants' tacit knowledge, enabling reflection and strengthening awareness of safe holistic practice [4]. This is in contrast to the teacher-centered approach of instruction, where the focus is on the knowledgeable teacher conveying information to those less knowledgeable [5]. While those conducting health simulations are frequently required to engage in both techniques, the focus of this chapter is on the attributes of the facilitator and process of facilitation.

Multiple methods of facilitation are possible, and use of any particular method is dependent on the experience level of the participant(s), their learning needs and the expected learning outcomes. Rather than offering a 'standard' experience, those facilitating simulations need to be mindful of what people *bring*

Healthcare Simulation Education: Evidence, Theory and Practice, First Edition.
Edited by Debra Nestel, Michelle Kelly, Brian Jolly and Marcus Watson.
© 2018 John Wiley & Sons Ltd. Published 2018 by John Wiley & Sons Ltd.

to the situation [6]. Participants' level of knowledge, skills, attitudes, behaviours and experience of previous simulations, as well as other life experiences, are key considerations concerning the anticipated degree of facilitation required. We flag 'anticipated' as a qualifier due to the unintended and opportunistic nature of learning that emerges during simulations, which may not always align with the facilitator's perspective of the degree of support required or, equally, what participants *should* gain from the experience [7].

Attributes of a facilitator

One of the key attributes of a simulation facilitator is that of establishing and maintaining an environment of trust. Trust is essential to foster a psychologically safe learning environment, one in which actions and thought processes can be analysed to reiterate appropriate performance or to highlight areas requiring improvement [3]. Facilitators must be able to take note of and interpret participants' visual and auditory responses during the simulation, and to present key points for discussion during the debrief [3, 4, 8]. An approach of inclusiveness, coordinating and directing an engaging dialogue, particularly during the debriefing, is one of the most challenging aspects of facilitation. The attributes of a skilled facilitator include awareness of techniques that stimulate participants' independent responses, and ways of raising mindfulness to elicit reflection, while being attentive to cultural diversity, norms and differing expectations of engagement [8]. Illustrations of how the attributes of the facilitator contribute to the simulation learning experience are captured in this chapter.

The process of facilitation

In reference to the NHET-Sim model (see Chapter 18), the process of facilitating simulations is multilayered and interconnected. Facilitation commences with conceptualization and planning of the briefing, strategies for facilitating the activity itself, the important debriefing/feedback session, through to the reflection and evaluation stages. Examples of processes for facilitating simulations in each of these phases are provided in what follows.

Conceptualization

At a conceptual level, understanding the overarching purpose and goal of simulation activity is fundamental. The goals of a particular scenario are often represented as learning objectives and outcomes with which the activity needs to align [9, 10]. However, we argue that there is an additional need to consider a conceptual approach to simulation facilitation that is consistent with the pedagogical framework of the curriculum or aims of continuing education programs. Examples of such frameworks include problem or inquiry-based learning [11, 12], clinical reasoning [13] and clinical judgement [6], which in essence promote experience-based learning inclusive of reflection. Conceptualization should take into account the level of higher-order thinking represented in the learning outcomes, the degree of facilitation anticipated during the simulation and the model of debriefing. The overall intent is to highlight the connectedness between what is being simulated and how the learning, and reflection, might be assimilated into participants' knowledge frameworks about individual practice. Triggering participants to think about and reflect on practice is the core intent of the facilitation process. Probing, open-ended questions and nuanced guidance help to achieve this aim.

Aligning simulation activities with the pedagogical frameworks of a curriculum or program, we believe, is integral to informing the level of facilitation and the role of the facilitator. Support for this belief exists in the ways in which carefully considered guidance provided by the facilitator is valued even by final-year nursing students as an important component of simulation practice, in facilitating understanding through application and evaluation of critical thinking and clinical judgement [14].

Simulations should complement adequate theoretical and procedural content to ensure that learners or participants have a schema, or mental model, to contextualize ways of reacting and responding during a scenario. Similarly, simulations of specialist practice require an appropriate level of exposure, supported with explanation and exploration of more complex practices. When simulations are scheduled as preparation for upcoming clinical experiences [15], students have reported benefit in having sufficient time following the simulation to reflect on their performances or make sense of what they have observed, in order to fine-tune their practice [16, 17]. These higher-level concepts are important: to position the simulations within and across curricula or programs and plan for the level of support and facilitation that adequately scaffolds students' learning.

Planning for facilitation

The role of the facilitator, and of facilitation, can be critical to participants' simulation experience. Facilitation is most commonly represented in the literature as an element of the post-simulation debrief. However, an understanding of facilitation and the need to consider the role of the facilitator as part of simulation design are of great importance to ensure that the learning and learners' experience of simulation are as intended.

Being a simulation facilitator requires multiple faces, many of them invisible. Hellaby [18] notes that a simulation facilitator is often expected to have many roles, such as providing guiding cues or prompts; juggling technological and equipment issues; setting up the simulation environment; providing information to improve realism; and conducting a debrief. In other words, the role of the facilitator is one of support, structure and guidance. Aspects of the simulation environment, the technical complexity of the equipment and the artifacts or materials with which participants can interact during scenarios all contribute to the ways in which simulations can be facilitated. The ideal situation would be to have support from technical or laboratory personnel to manage some of these elements while the facilitator focuses on the unfolding action from an educational perspective.

Planning for facilitation requires thinking about the potential strategies required to guide participants through the simulation. Such strategies need careful consideration due to the unpredictability of participants' responses, or unexpected technical disruptions, during the simulation. Rehearsing the simulation scenario is highly recommended, to test the scenario for timing and whether the roles enable enough action or participation, and to validate the applicability and strength of the scenario topic for the intended group.

Where there is perceived to be mixed enthusiasm within groups, role allocation may be challenging. To keep the simulation action moving along, it may be necessary deliberately to select participants for specific roles, particularly where leadership is a component of a role. Engagement of all students in the action of the simulation is an important aim, and in Australia where large student groups are commonplace, maximizing the interest of those who observe simulations is an area attracting interest. Ultimately, when talking about strategies for facilitating participants' progression through a simulation, we are talking about cues.

Level of feedback and cueing

Cues have been defined as responses of actions that offer just enough information for participants to progress through a simulation activity, but do not interfere with their thought processes [19]. Research exploring cues and cueing as a designed characteristic of simulation planning categorizes these as *conceptual* or *reality* cues [20]. Conceptual cues provide a kind of instructional support that assists participant progression in the form of adequate information or feedback [20]. The source of such feedback may include monitoring equipment (changes to the ECG), a comment from the patient (the pain is very different from anything I've had before) or the information included on patient notes (nitrate spray ordered as PRN medication) [21]. Reality cues are designed elements of a simulation that overcome the shortcomings of a simulator or a simulation to reflect real life [20]. Reality cues may include the facilitator handing a 12-lead echogardiograph printout showing ST changes indicative of myocardial ischaemia, or a printed statement posted to the mannequin's feet stating 'feet are warm and dry'.

Important considerations for cues and cueing include the authentic ways in which information or feedback would be encountered in real practice [20, 22]. Determining a patient's fluid balance may involve an assortment of beverages at the bedside, or a indwelling urinary catheter containing a deliberate volume of concentrated urine to infer dehydration. Information can also be communicated to participants from confederates or through the voice of the mannequin. Confederates (as distinct from simulated patients, see Chapter 10) can be scripted into a simulation to enhance realism, provide challenges and augment the educational integrity of the activity by contributing additional information [23]. Confederates can provide tacit cues and prompts such as tone of voice, eye contact and body language, and these may provide a focus for understanding the ill-defined social and cultural elements of engaging with people.

Confederates may adopt the role of family, healthcare professionals or bystanders, guiding the progression of the simulation but not playing a central role within the simulation [23–25]. While confederates may be educators, clinicians, researchers, actors or students, adequate preparation is required to ensure that their intended purposes of guiding learners, facilitating a safe environment, contributing to the realism of the simulation and providing a bridge between learners and the learning process are achieved [23].

Planning for facilitation also needs to balance carefully the replication of reality with a simulation experience that will facilitate learning. A commonly identified objective in the design of a healthcare simulation is to achieve a high degree of fidelity or realism, enabling participants to *suspend disbelief*, a state in which they believe that they are engaged in an experience that closely resembles real life [26, 27]. However, depending on participants' level of experience, the context being simulated and the learning outcomes underpinning the simulation, a highly realistic replica of a real practice environment may be unnecessary or may in fact impede learning through cognitive overload [28].

Planning for facilitation also requires consideration of the role of the facilitator. Will the facilitator play an active part in the simulation? Will learning be affected if participants are hesitant in their roles due to interacting with the facilitator? Exploring the true impact on learning when the facilitator is a collaborator in knowledge construction would enlighten and inform simulation practices. Such considerations are particularly pertinent for undergraduate nursing students, where perceptions of authority and knowledgeability can influence students' engagement, participation and the fidelity of the experience [29].

Facilitating large groups

The extent and type of facilitation will be dependent on the resources, personnel, number of participants and overall cohort size. A particular challenge when planning for facilitation of undergraduate nursing programs in Australia is the large number of participants. Challenges exist in terms of how to provide a meaningful simulation experience for large groups, as well as how to ensure a consistent experience if multiple facilitators are required. The steps detailed in Table 19.1 and Figure 19.1 provide strategies that one

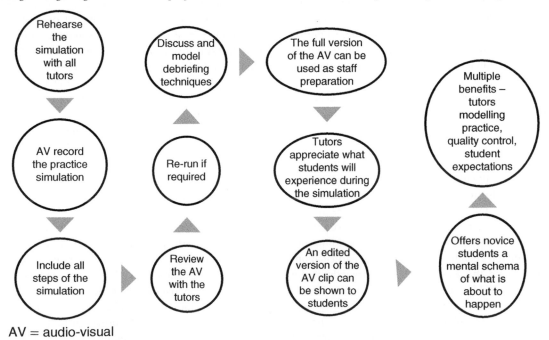

AV = audio-visual

Figure 19.1 Strategies for facilitating simulation with large numbers of tutors and novice students.

Table 19.1 Strategies for planning and delivering simulation for large student cohorts.

Strategy	Notes
Schedule a set time period (a full week) per semester for simulation within the curriculum.	A designated time for simulation can be quarantined within each semester. This type of learning experience is then identified as different to usual laboratory classes.
Determine a workable number of students per simulation session: a group of 10 or 12 students, for example, where half the group participate in the simulation while the other half observe. The halves then swap over.	Smaller group sizes enable a more intimate experience. Students can experience active and observer roles – and provide input to the debriefing discussions.
Structure a preparatory session, e.g. a skill refresher, just prior to the simulation session.	A skill refresher immediately prior to the simulation focuses learners on the skills likely to be required in the simulation. It aims to reduce anxiety and center students' attention on what is happening within the simulation.
In this example each session is 90 minutes, which equals 3 hours' combined simulation activity. This 'unit' is identified as 1 time cycle.	
The 'units' can be scalable depending on facilities and personnel. We have doubled the number of 'units' per time cycle to offer simulation to 20–24 students.	Other subjects/units/courses that occur during Simweek are moved to online mode to free up physical spaces.
Between 5 and 6 time cycles can be accommodated per day, including breaks for staff. A 3-hour simulation experience is thus achieved for 100–120 students per day.	The schedule addresses the pragmatics and tensions of providing a supported simulation experience for novice students according to contemporary practices, with the challenge of managing large numbers.
Over 5 days, 500–600 students can be cycled through simulation.	

Australian university has employed to address such challenges. These strategies have been used with novice student cohorts of between 450 and 600 people, and facilitator numbers ranging from 8 to 14, to ensure a consistent level of quality and experience for students [17, 30].

Where there are numerous facilitators, agreement must be reached beforehand on the types of cues and what kind of actions would trigger a 'pause and discuss' moment during the actual simulation. Strategies to be used for facilitating debriefing also need to be agreed and rehearsed beforehand. An audio-visual (AV) clip demonstrating the expected debriefing approach to be adopted may be useful in this regard (Figure 19.1). Despite the best efforts to maximize the number of active roles within a scenario, substantial numbers of students end up being observers.

Observers may be located within the simulation space or in an adjacent room viewing the live AV feed. They gain benefit from watching what unfolds and relating the scenario and activities to their own experience [14, 31]. Efforts have been made to maximize observer engagement through using checklists, for example in scenarios about resuscitation skills [32] or patient interview techniques [33]. Rubrics have also been used to elicit thoughts and feedback about clinical judgement. It is worth exploring options in this space, but the key is to prepare the observers for their tasks and contribution to discussions.

Briefing

Briefing (also referred to as pre-briefing) is described in some detail in Chapter 18. While there are a number of frequently cited elements to include in the briefing, sequencing is important. Appropriate sequencing aims to broadly capture the attention of participants, then to progressively focus their attention to the simulation.

Commencing the briefing by establishing the simulation 'ground-rules' not only sets the scene for an environment of dignity and mutual respect, but promotes a learning environment of psychological safety [34]. Vocalizing the learning outcomes orientates participants to the purpose of the simulation and helps focus attention. Orientating the active players to the simulated setting is important to ensure familiarity with the resources available and their location, and also provides an opportunity to negotiate differences between the simulation environment and the 'real world' and to reduce anxiety [35].

If engaging with a simulator is integral to the scenario, ensure that participants have an opportunity to practise the skills that will be required (for example obtaining a blood pressure, auscultating lung fields). For participants who are new to simulation, one useful strategy is to include a skills review session (see Table 19.1) or to play a short video clip of the pending simulation (Figure 19.1). These combined elements help learners focus on the psychomotor skills that might be required of them in the simulation, to build a schema about ways of interacting during the scenario, with the overall intent of developing professional behaviours [36, 37]. This approach balances the need for providing novice students with adequate information around the upcoming, new experience while maintaining a level of spontaneity in responses to the simulation scenario.

Briefing should also include information about the duration of the scenario, how participants will know the simulation has commenced and, importantly (but often neglected), how participants will know it has ended. Providing the patient handover to participants is one strategy that indicates the transition from briefing to the simulation scenario. The handover offers context for the simulation experience, focuses and prepares participants for learning and represents real-world practice. How much information to provide is an important consideration. The patient handover, as with much of the briefing, provides cues designed to facilitate learning. Too little information and participants may have insufficient cues to anticipate what is expected of them. Too many cues in the form of a long handover risks participants being overwhelmed. A useful strategy is to provide the patient handover to those actively participating in the simulation in both verbal and written forms, to refer to during the scenario if required.

From this definitive starting point, the options and approaches to facilitation *during* the simulation activity will now be discussed. As indicated from the outset, the methods of facilitation described can be adapted for other health disciplines and learners, and the level of support will vary according to participant expertise and how the simulation scenario unfolds.

Facilitating the simulation activity

Allocating roles to participants may appear an easy task, but the anxiety that surrounds performing in front of others, uncertainty in what is about to unfold or the expectations of the participant can influence this aspect of simulation. Allowing novice students to work

in pairs to share the decision making offers a level of peer support. Whichever strategies are used – and benefits can be argued for either self-selection or tutor allocation – assisting participants to 'get into role' is an important responsibility of the facilitator. Clinical props such as disposable gowns with name tags to identify each person's role help participants remember who is who, and also orientate the observers so that they can track team members and interactions. For those assuming the role of a relative, civilian clothes, wigs or spectacles can help with immersion into that role.

As the simulation scenario unfolds, the anticipated direction of the learning activity can be guided in a number of ways: through the voice of the mannequin; via a confederate or simulated patient; or at a simplistic level by the facilitator, who may be at the periphery of the room. There are differing opinions about whether the facilitator should assume one of the roles in the simulation, since students may be fear doing or saying the 'wrong' thing. From experience, if the scenario incorporates complex clinical procedures, and students need to learn how to assist with such techniques, there is justification for a facilitator taking an active role.

There is much debate about whether to interrupt a scenario. Essentially, we believe that there are no hard-and-fast rules here. If the momentum of a simulation is waning, interrupting and resetting the direction is more important than letting novice students struggle in knowing how to respond. Similarly, where participants venture into unplanned domains or overact, it would be best to end the simulation and follow up on these aspects in the debriefing or separately with the individual(s) afterwards.

As mentioned earlier, harnessing the perspectives of those observing the simulation action is an area that is gaining interest. There are various ways of enabling observer engagement in simulations. In essence, providing targeted questions for them to address about what they see, or allocating people to focus on the actions of a particular participant, can add another dimension to the debriefing discussions.

Knowing when to conclude the simulation is an equally important part of facilitation. Some facilitators may continue the scenario until the learning objectives have been met. Time constraints may determine the end of a scenario. Often the simulation action will reach a natural conclusion, at which time a statement such as 'end of the simulation' should be clearly voiced.

As simulations elicit the emotional aspects of learning, helping participants to get out of role is as important as helping them get into role.

The use of AV recording systems appears to have waned in recent years. It would be challenging to facilitate a simulation as well as view the unfolding scenario and tag or log events on an AV recording. Ideally, an additional person should manage the AV tasks to ensure that the facilitator can fulfil their responsibilities without distraction. The additional time required to use AV playback in the debriefing may not be possible given time constraints (particularly with large groups). However, AV playback, particularly for self-debriefing or peer debriefing, is a popular strategy and can contribute to reflection of and about practice. Caution needs to be exercised about the distribution and unintended use of AV materials beyond the simulation event. The majority of simulation centers that regularly use AV recordings in simulation delete the material immediately after the event.

Facilitating debriefing, providing feedback and triggering reflection

There are a range of frameworks that could be used to debrief participants following simulations and more detailed discussion of techniques is accommodated elsewhere in this book (see Chapter 21), so only an overview of important elements in relation to the facilitation of simulations is offered here. In essence, the intent of the debriefing or feedback session is to draw comments from the participants about their recollections and opinions about how the scenario played out, and areas that may need attention in future practice. Setting the environment for the discussion (reminding people of the intent, positioning the active participants and the observer group) can considerably influence how this session unfolds.

How the facilitator conducts the debrief is one of the most important aspects of this role. Critical components in triggering reflection and learning during debriefing are for the facilitator to use open-ended questions; prompt for more information; aim to encourage all participants to voice their opinions about the scenario events; and connect the scenario actions and outcomes with the relevance of clinical practices. Being comfortable with periods of silence during debriefing is

important to master – participants will inevitably feel compelled to break the silence with a contribution. Incorporating comments from the observers enables a level of peer review and a sense of community. Approaches to amplify the engagement of observers with specific contributions to the debriefing form an area of current interest and investigation [38]. As Rooney et al. advocate [4], creating agile observers in simulation may lead to agile observers and learners in clinical practice. Orchestrating the debriefing to take account of all these viewpoints requires a level of expertise. However, creating the opportunity to discuss what was observed in the simulation, bring to light the thought processes behind the actions and intertwining opinions from peers most often lead to a situation of enlightenment about practice.

Further work is being undertaken in this area to generate observer learning and feedback in the debriefing about the all-encompassing, holistic elements of practice [4, 38].

Evaluation of facilitation

In recognition of the important role that a facilitator plays in learning through simulation, feedback about the facilitation process is becoming an important feature. Evaluation can be sourced from participants, peers and through self-reflection (drawing on AV footage). As frequently demonstrated, one's own opinion about perceived performance can either contradict or corroborate how others view things. Refining facilitation techniques and seeing the impact on engagement and learning can be equally rewarding for the facilitator.

Conclusion

There are a variety of approaches to facilitating healthcare simulations. The approach depends on participants' level of expertise and what they bring to the situation; the simulation learning objectives and intended outcomes; and how the scenario and expected participant responses play out. Similarly, the experience and attributes of the facilitator shape how they conduct and respond to events during and following the simulation.

Facilitating simulations spans more than just the activity, and should incorporate the elements of conceptualization, preparation, briefing, the activity and debriefing through to reflection and evaluation. Strategies for ensuring a quality experience for students when managing large numbers of facilitators, and techniques to assist participants through the phases of a simulation, have been raised in this chapter.

References

1 Nestel, D. and Bearman, M. (2015) Theory and simulation-based education: definitions, worldviews and applications. *Clin Simul Nurs*, **11** (8), 349–54.

2 Franklin, A.E., Boese, T., Gloe, D. *et al.* (2011) Standards of best practice: Simulation Standard IV: Facilitation. *Clin Simul Nurs*, **2** (6 Suppl), s19–s21.

3 Boese, T., Cato, M., Gonzalez, L. *et al.* (2013) Standards of best practice: Simulation Standard V: Facilitator. *Clin Simul Nurs*, **9** (6S), s22–s25.

4 Rooney, D., Hopwood, N., Boud, D. and Kelly, M.A. (2015) The role of simulation in pedagogies of higher education for the health professions: through a practice-based lens. *Vocat Learn*, **8** (3), 269–85.

5 Dismukes, R.K., McDonnell, L.K., Jobe, K.K. and Smith, G.M. (2000) What is facilitation and why use it? in *Facilitation and debriefing in aviation training and operations. Studies in aviation psychology and human factors* (eds R.K. Dismukes and G.M. Smith), Ashgate, Aldershot, pp. 1–12.

6 Tanner, C. (2006) Thinking like a nurse: a research-based model of clinical judgment in nursing. *J Nurs Educ*, **45** (6), 204–21.

7 Kelly, M.A. and Hager, P. (2015) Informal learning: relevance and application to health care simulation. *Clin Simul Nurs*, **11** (8), 376–82.

8 Chung, H.S., Dieckmann, P. and Issenberg, S.B. (2013) It is time to consider cultural differences in debriefing. *Simul Healthc*, **8** (3), 166–70.

9 Lioce, L., Reed, C.C., Lemon, D. *et al.* (2013) Standards of best practice: Simulation Standard III: Participant objectives. *Clin Simul Nurs*, **9** (6S), s15–s18.

10 Arthur, C., Levett-Jones, T. and Kable, A. (2013) Quality indicators for the design and implementation of simulation experiences: a Delphi study. *Nurs Educ Today*, **33** (11), 1357–61.

11 Cleverly, D. (2003) *Implementing inquiry-based learning in nursing*, Routledge, New York.

12 Clouston, T. (2010) *Problem based learning in health and social care*, Wiley, Hoboken, NJ.

13 Levett-Jones, T. (ed.) (2013) *Clinical reasoning: learning to think like a nurse*, Pearson, Sydney.

14 Kelly, M.A., Hager, P. and Gallagher, R. (2014) What matters most? Students' rankings of simulation components which contribute to clinical judgement. *J Nurs Educ*, **53** (2), 97–101.

15 Doerr, H. and Bosseau, M.W. (2008) How to build a successful simulation strategy: the simulation learning pyramid, in *Clinical simulation: operations, engineering and management* (eds R. Kyle and W. Murray), Elsevier, New York.

16 Kable, A.K., Arthur, C., Levett-Jones, T. and Reid-Searl, K. (2013) Student evaluation of simulation in undergraduate nursing programs in Australia using quality indicators. *Nurs Health Sci*, **15** (2), 235–43.

17 Disler, R., Rochester, S., Kelly, M.A. *et al.* (2013) Delivering a large cohort simulation: beginning nursing students' experience: a pre-post survey. *J Nurs Educ Pract*, **3** (12), 133–42.

18 Hellaby, M. (2013) *Healthcare simulation in practice*, M&K Publishing, Keswick.

19 Jeffries, P.R. and Rogers, K.J. (2007) Theoretical framework for simulation design, in *Simulation in nursing education: from conceptualization to evaluation* (ed. P.R. Jeffries), National League for Nursing, New York, pp. 21–33.

20 Paige, J.B. and Morin, K.H. (2013) Simulation fidelity and cueing: a systematic review of the literature. *Clin Simul Nurs*, **9** (11), e481–e489.

21 Motola, I., Devine, L.A., Chung, H.S., Sullivan, J.E., Issenberg, S.B. Simulation in healthcare education: a best evidence practical guide. AMEE Guide No. 82. *Med Teach*. 2013;**35**(10):e1511–e1530. PubMed PMID: 23941678.

22 Dieckmann, P., Manser, T., Wehner, T. and Rall, M. (2007) Reality and fiction cues in medical patient simulation: an interview study with anesthesiologists. *J Cogn Eng Decis Mak*, **1** (2), 148–68.

23 Nestel, D., Mobley, B.L., Hunt, E.A. and Eppich, W.J. (2014) Confederates in health care simulations: not as simple as it seems. *Clin Simul Nurs*, **10** (12), 611–16.

24 Gloe, D., Sando, C.R., Franklin, A.E. *et al.* (2013) Standards of best practice: Simulation Standard II: Professional integrity of participant(s). *Clin Simul Nurs*, **9** (6 Suppl), s12–s14.

25 Meakim, C., Boese, T., Decker, S. *et al.* (2013) Standards of best practice: Simulation Standard I: Terminology. *Clin Simul Nurs*, **9** (6 Suppl), s3–s11.

26 Seropian, M.A., Brown, J.S., Gavilanes, J.S. and Driggers, B. (2004) Simulation: not just a manikin. *J Nurs Educ*, **43** (4), 164–6.

27 Dieckmann, P., Gaba, D. and Rall, M. (2007) Deepening the theoretical foundations of patient simulation as social practice. *Simul Healthc*, **2** (3), 183–93.

28 Van Merriënboer, J.J.G. and Sweller, J. (2010) Cognitive load theory in health professional education: design principles and strategies. *Med Educ*, **44** (1), 85–93.

29 Jeong S.Y, Hickey N, Levett-Jones, T. et al. Understanding and enhancing the learning experiences of culturally and linguistically diverse nursing students in an Australian bachelor of nursing program. *Nurs Educ Today*. 2011;**31**(3):238–44. PubMed PMID: 21078536.

30 Rochester, S., Kelly, M.A., Disler, R. *et al.* (2012) Providing simulation experiences for large cohorts of 1st year nursing students: evaluating quality and impact. *Collegian*, **19** (3), 117–24.

31 Levett-Jones, T., Andersen, P., Reid-Searl, K. *et al.* (2015) Tag team simulation: an innovative approach for promoting active engagement of participants and observers during group simulations. *Nurs Educ Pract*, **15** (5), 345–52.

32 Dilley, S.J, Weiland, T.J, O'Brien, R. et al. Use of a checklist during observation of a simulated cardiac arrest scenario does not improve time to CPR and defibrillation over observation alone for subsequent scenarios. *Teach Learn Med*. 2015;**27**(1):71–9. PubMed PMID: 25584474.

33 Sennekamp, M., Gilbert, K., Gerlach, F.M., Guethlin, C. Development and validation of the 'FrOCK': Frankfurt observer communication checklist. *Zeitschrift fur Evidenz, Fortbildung und Qualitat im Gesundheitswesen.* 2012;**106**(8):595–601. PubMed PMID: 23084867.

34 Rudolph, J.W., Raemer, D.B. and Simon, R. (2014) Establishing a safe container for learning in simulation: the role of the presimulation briefing. *Simul Healthc*, **9** (6), 339–49.

35 INACSL Board of Directors (2011) Standard IV: Facilitation methods. *Clin Simul Nurs*, **35** (4, Suppl), S12–S13.

36 Berragan, L. (2011) Simulation: an effective pedagogical approach for nursing? *Nurs Educ Today*, **31** (7), 660–63.

37 McNiesh, S.G. (2015) Cultural norms of clinical simulation in undergraduate nursing education. *Glob Qual Nurs Res.*, **2**, 1–10.

38 O'Regan, S., Watterson, L. and Nestel, D. (in press) Observer roles in healthcare simulation: a systematic review. *Adv Simul.*

CHAPTER 20

Strategies for managing adverse events in healthcare simulations

Stuart Marshall & Cate McIntosh

KEY MESSAGES

- Most adverse events in simulation are amenable to prevention by attention to good design or thorough preparation, or both.

- Adverse events may be categorized as physical, psychological and those related to transfer of learning.

- Programmes require strategies to prevent and manage learning-related, physical and psychological adverse events.

Overview

This chapter will examine what happens when simulations do not go to plan. This may vary from unexpected distractions to events that cause harm to participants and staff. We will discuss the key importance of preparation in preventing these adverse events and strategies for managing them when they arise. Topics include learner preparation, environmental safety (electrical safety, sharps), psychological counselling to minimize distress, dealing with real clinical events (chest pain, strokes) and with egregious performance (legal and moral obligations, disclosure).

Introduction

One of the inherent characteristics of simulation-based education is the low risk presented to patients. However, despite the best intentions of educators, events with potential for physical or psychological harm to learners, educators or even patients do occasionally arise. Effective design, thorough planning including development of contingency plans and preparation of learners are key to preventing and mitigating any harm caused. Simulation educators should be familiar with local policies and procedures to manage emergencies if they do occur. Strategies should be in place to learn from adverse events related to simulation and to prevent future similar events. This chapter outlines the preparation that should occur to prevent harm from simulation, and discusses sources of physical and psychological injury and how they may be managed.

Adverse events in simulation

For the purposes of this chapter, adverse events in simulation can be loosely categorized as follows:
- Learning related adverse events
  a. No learning occurs
  b. Learning occurs but transfer fails (i.e. unable to put into practice what has been learnt)
  c. Transfer occurs but the practice is applied inappropriately (wrong time, wrong situation, omissions of essential steps). This 'negative transfer' may lead to near misses in the clinical environment or actual harm to patients
- Physical adverse events
  a. Injury to learners (e.g. sharps injury)
  b. Injury to staff (e.g. attempting to defibrillate an actor)
  c. Failure to recognize actual clinical events
- Psychological adverse events
  a. Acute distress
  b. Post-traumatic stress disorder

Healthcare Simulation Education: Evidence, Theory and Practice, First Edition.
Edited by Debra Nestel, Michelle Kelly, Brian Jolly and Marcus Watson.
© 2018 John Wiley & Sons Ltd. Published 2018 by John Wiley & Sons Ltd.

Preparation of learners

The primary method of preventing adverse events related to simulation is by preparation of the learners. This includes attention to good instructional design (Chapter 2), making the physical environment safe and psychologically preparing the learners to participate in the simulation. In fact, to some extent the term 'unexpected' events is a misnomer, since most adverse events in simulation are due to either poor design or poor preparation, or both.

Being explicit about expectations and pointing out potential dangers during a familiarization and briefing process is important to prevent physical injury, for instance from attempts to move a heavy mannequin. When dealing with very junior clinicians, these instructions may need to address as yet unfamiliar issues such as safe disposal of sharps and electrical safety.

Psychological preparation of learners is also important, starting with an introduction to the session and the facility. Learners are often nervous and unsure of what to expect from a simulation encounter. Giving learners an opportunity to express this and reassuring them that it is normal may help relieve some anxiety. The purpose of the session should be made clear. If the session is for purely formative educational purposes, it should be made explicit that no testing or feedback to employers or supervisors will occur. If the purpose is assessment, the expectations for how that will proceed should be clarified.

Familiarization with the simulation environment helps reduce anxiety by giving learners an opportunity to examine the room in which they will be working and to understand what is expected of them. In a study of 11 junior nurses attending their first simulation session, the familiarization process helped reduce levels of unpleasant emotions while maintaining activation and readiness to learn [1]. The introductory and familiarization components set the tone for the rest of the simulation course. Additional skills sessions, revision of key materials and an opportunity to ask questions are important to give learners the tools they need to succeed in any immersive simulation scenario.

Preparing a safe physical environment

A simulation environment should conform to the safety standards of the facility in which it is located. In many regards the preparation of a safe simulation environment is as clear-cut as the preparation of a safe clinical environment; the equipment and functions are broadly the same and thus many of the occupational health and safety (OH&S) considerations are similar. For example, storage of gas cylinders and gas delivery systems must conform to local standards; testing and maintenance of electrical supplies must be ensured; and manual-handling requirements should be observed. The design of simulation facilities should take into account the local building codes to prevent injuries caused by dangerous electrical, gas or water plumbing issues. Designers specializing in the development of clinical and simulation facilities should be engaged whenever possible.

There are a number of differences from the clinical setting that are of note, however.

Electrical devices

In clinical settings processes exist for the testing of clinical equipment. The use in simulation of old or expired equipment that may no longer be serviced could lead to electrical hazards. A routine programme of basic electrical safety checks is required for all equipment used in simulation, even if there is no intent for it to be used on patients.

Defibrillators

Defibrillators require specific mention due to the higher frequency of use in simulation settings and potential for injury. Learners, particularly novices, using defibrillators may be unfamiliar with the safety procedures to prevent injury. These may include musculoskeletal injuries or life-threatening arrhythmias caused by contact with the patient or metal object during the defibrillation shock. Many centres opt to have the defibrillators modified such that the electrical current is absent or minimal, although this may be expensive and requires a skilled biomedical engineer. Another option is to have the electrical energy 'absorbed' by a proprietary device before it reaches the mannequin.

Fluids

Care should be taken with any fluids around electrical equipment. In particular, substantial and expensive damage can occur to mannequins should fluid be spilled on them. Learners should be made aware of this and requested to inform an instructor should this occur, and to move away from the mannequin or device to avoid an electrical shock. Fluids should also be drained from mannequins at the end of the session to prevent damage to circuitry and/or growth of mildew in hard-to-access locations.

Gas supplies

Compressed air can be used as a substitute for many gases when building a simulation facility, but some mannequins and devices may require oxygen, nitrous oxide, carbon dioxide and/or nitrogen. Care must be taken to prevent sparks and fires in the presence of oxidizing gases such as oxygen and nitrous oxide. Real anaesthetic agents may also be used that require scavenging from the simulation room. Provision of actual carbon dioxide in an anaesthetic scenario through a standard absorbent circuit led to the near-miss of an overheated canister in one case report that could potentially have burned a staff member or student [2]. Compressors used for the running of mannequins need to be bled after use and require regular servicing to ensure safe use.

Mannequins

There is a risk of fire when live defibrillators are used in oxygen-enriched environments, for example when a defibrillator is attached to a mannequin being ventilated with oxygen. Before connecting devices to mannequins, always ensure that there are no safety implications by reading the manufacturer's instructions and safety alerts [3]. There are currently no recorded cases of mannequin fires, but many centres now consider it good practice to use *either* a live defibrillator *or* oxygen-enriched gases, but not both.

Sharps injuries

Failure to make expectations clear, failure to provide an appropriate safety briefing for junior learners, and failure to adhere to good sharps-handling practice (e.g. resheathing sharps to 'save money') poses a risk to participants and staff. Processes such as sharps disposal should be reinforced and an expectation must be set that everyone will practise as safely as possible in simulation and clinical work.

Drugs and other clinical supplies

Programmes should have a clear policy on the use of real versus simulated drugs and clinical supplies. Use of real drugs and supplies requires attention to any inherent physical risks such as sharps, chemical irritation and spills. Containing expired drugs and supplies to the simulation facility or area is important to prevent mixing of 'real' supplies with simulation supplies.

Virtual and other display devices

The use of advanced displays and virtual reality devices is currently rare in healthcare. However, the expansion of three-dimensional (3D) displays for surgery and the availability of products like Oculus Rift (see Chapter 10) are likely to introduce new challenges for physical safety. Virtual reality (VR), augmented reality, 3D displays (screens and cave automatic virtual environments) have the potential to induce simulator sickness (also known as cyber-sickness and VR sickness). If using this equipment, simulation programmes should have appropriate simulator sickness minimization and response strategies.

In situ simulation

Simulation in the clinical environment carries substantial additional risks [4]. Centers conducting in situ simulations should have clearly described policies describing the management of drugs, equipment and supplies to avoid putting patients at risk. Careful consideration should be given as to whether expired drugs or supplies are brought into the clinical environment and to which equipment is to be used during the simulation. Patients have in the past inadvertently received non-sterile water as intravenous fluid, with serious outcomes [5]. Using real clinical supplies or equipment may mean that the equipment is not available should an actual emergency arise or that unrecognized contamination occurs, such as with the de-sterilization of surgical equipment.

Confederates and SPs

Clear expectations should be communicated with participants about the roles and actions of any actors in the scenario, for example to prevent inadvertent needle-stick injuries of actors in situations that would normally require intravenous cannulation.

Preparing a safe psychological 'container' for learning

Serious psychological harm such as post-traumatic stress disorder (PTSD) is thought to be rare in participants.

More common psychological disturbances include acute anxiety, depression and rumination over the events of the simulation. More damaging responses may manifest as an avoidance of situations in the clinical setting and reliving of the simulation experience several weeks or months after the event. These serious reactions may indicate the onset of PTSD.

Much of the psychological safety of the learners to prevent adverse reactions is created in the initial introduction and familiarization stages, as already noted. Rudolph et al. [6] describe four ways of safeguarding learners from adverse psychological harm: clarifying what is expected of learners; agreement that learners will treat the scenarios as real (often termed a 'fiction contract'); showing participants how to get things done in the simulation setting; and showing respect for learners and their psychological safety.

Debriefing is perhaps the most vulnerable time for participants. It is important that the expectations are restated prior to the debriefing and that overly critical and unhelpful comments from other participants are prevented, moderated and put into context for any exposed participants.

Occasionally unforeseen circumstances arise, such as a traumatic neonatal resuscitation triggering memories of a recent event that a participant has encountered in their clinical work. Rarely, the simulation triggers memory of more personal events such as the loss of a child, spouse or relative. It is of course impossible to predict whether participants will have adverse responses to scenarios, but it is essential to ensure that they feel supported by the faculty through the course. The role of a secondary debriefer includes looking for signs of distress in the participant group such as body language signals, for instance lack of eye contact or withdrawal from the discussion. Upset participants should be dealt with on an individual basis; that is, there is no one right way to manage an upset participant. Their emotions should not be ignored and some people may respond well to a gentle offer to discuss their feelings during the debriefing. Others may prefer a private discussion afterwards. A participant leaving a debriefing in an upset state requires follow-up by one of the faculty. In addition, it is important to check in with people who have shown signs of distress before they leave at the end of the day. Some simulation services provide access to external psychological counselling if participants consider that the issues experienced during the simulations have not been resolved.

Psychological safety is also important for the educators, as events may also trigger unpleasant memories and experiences for members of the instructor team. Acting out events following a personal incident requires similar support for the educator from their colleagues.

Death of the 'patient'

Certain simulations are designed to explore breaking bad news or end-of-life issues. Great care should be taken to respect the learners and their emotional well-being if this is planned. It is usually appropriate in these circumstances to explain prior to the scenario, or immediately afterwards, that the patient will die or that the patient could not be saved irrespective of the actions of the participants. Even with the knowledge that it was planned, participants may still reflect poorly on their performance and be overly self-critical. It should be identified that these are high-risk scenarios for the development of adverse responses, particularly in those learners that have experienced recent grief. Recent evidence shows a substantial increase in the stress response of participants when a simulation death occurs [7], which may require additional resources as routine. Provision of a separate, independent psychologist or counsellor at the time of the scenario or their contact details afterwards is advised.

Real clinical events

Actual events unrelated to the simulation can and do still occur in simulation settings. Participants or staff may be taken ill and require medical attention. Simulation programmes should have a clearly articulated local policy and procedure for dealing with medical emergencies, including how help is summoned and how to communicate 'this is not a simulation!' or 'this is a real clinical event'. Facilities need to agree on specific language to communicate this in the event that help needs to be summoned. For example, industries that perform emergency testing such as fire-response systems use the term 'no duff'. All participants and staff should be familiarized with this policy at the start of a session. Medical assistance should be sought from outside the simulation facility if required by the local emergency response mechanism. Isolation of simulation equipment should occur, such that no equipment intended for simulation reaches the injured staff member or participant. Similarly, fire evacuation and alerting procedures should be followed and the participants briefed on these at the beginning of the session.

It is recommended that each centre have its own set of emergency procedures. These procedures may be developed in conjunction with broader organizational policies.

Legal and moral obligations of centres

Simulation professionals have a moral obligation to ensure the safety of not only the staff and participants within the centre but also, albeit indirectly, the patients served by these learners. Educators must ensure that they are up to date with the clinical guidelines they teach and that any dangerous behaviours observed in simulation are addressed appropriately. The absolute legal obligations differ between countries and jurisdictions, and these should be taken into account when writing protocols and procedures.

Recording and retention of data

Decisions about whether to record and/or retain audio-visual data will vary, depending on the nature of the learners and the purpose of the simulations. Irrespective of these considerations, all centres should have a clearly stated policy regarding the collection of audio-visual data, and all learners, staff and visitors should be informed of this policy.

Personal data such as attendance records that centres collected should be held according to the legal requirements of the local data protection legislation. These laws often have the provision for individuals to view their own data and these should be available if requested.

Data around personal performance and videos of participants in simulation are not 'discoverable' documents in many legal systems. Audio-visual data from simulations should not be released without the knowledge and written consent of all the individuals involved in the simulation. There may be exceptions to these situations, such as participants giving explicit consent for review of their performance for certification or research purposes.

Any data collected for research purposes should be handled according to the guidelines of the local Institutional Review Board. In general, this requires data to be kept in a secure location and destroyed after a specified time, typically five to seven years.

Reporting obligations

All educators and clinicians have a responsibility to report dangerous *clinical* behaviour by any health professional. However, simulation is not clinical practice; limitations in instructional design and technological limitations may cause learners to interpret cues in different ways, and consequently performance may not be representative of clinical practice. Dangerous behaviours should be addressed immediately with the learner in order to make an assessment about the nature of the lapse, so that misinterpretation of cues and performance gaps can be addressed during debriefing. If other learners, staff or simulated patients are considered to be at risk during the simulation, the scenario should be terminated. Depending on the extent and nature of the dangerous behaviour observed, it may also be necessary to discuss the performance with the learner after the session has concluded to determine other courses of action that may be required. These might include recommendations about additional learning opportunities or further discussions with supervisors or managers who can determine whether the behaviour forms part of a pattern that is also observed in clinical practice. In these cases, further performance assessment and workplace-based observation may be recommended or, in extreme cases, reporting may be considered.

Conclusion

The old adage 'an ounce of prevention is worth a pound of cure' should be kept in mind, since most adverse physical and psychological events can be prevented by adequate preparation of the learners and the environment. When events do occur, these must be mitigated early by the use of clear, pre-prepared guidelines and protocols. To fulfil our collective mission of optimizing patient care, simulation professionals have an obligation to their colleagues, to their learners and to their patients to ensure the safety and efficacy of simulation-based education.

References

1 Ballinger-Doran, S. (2010) *Preparation (familiarisation) of learners into the simulation-based learning environment. Master's of Education thesis*, Monash University, Melbourne.

2 Riem, N., Boet, S. and Chandra, D. (2011) Setting standards for simulation in anesthesia: the role of safety criteria in accreditation standards. *Can J Anesth.*, **58**, 846–52.

3 Laerdal (2015) *Safety notification: risk of fire with oxygen enriched environments*, Oakleigh, Laerdal Australia.

4 Patterson, M.D., Blike, G.T. and Nadkarni, V.M. (2008) In situ simulation: challenges and results, in *Advances in patient safety: new directions and alternative approaches, vol. 3: performance and tools* (eds K. Henriksen, J.B. Battles, M.A. Keyes and M.L. Grady), AHRQ, Rockville, MD.

5 FDA. FDA's investigation into patients being injected with simulated IV fluids continues [cited 14 September 2016]. Available at: http://www.fda.gov/Drugs/DrugSafety/ucm 428431.htm

6 Rudolph, J.W., Raemer, D.B. and Simon, R. (2014) Establishing a safe container for learning in simulation: the role of the presimulation briefing. *Simul Healthc.*, **9**, 339–49.

7 Goldberg, A., Silverman, E., Samuelson, S. *et al.* (2015) Learning through simulated independent practice leads to better future performance in a simulated crisis than learning through simulated supervised practice. *Br J Anaesth*, **114** (5), 794–800.

CHAPTER 21

Debriefing: The state of the art and science in healthcare simulation

Adam Cheng, Walter Eppich, Taylor Sawyer & Vincent Grant

KEY MESSAGES

- Debriefing conversations remain a cornerstone of effective simulation-based education.

- Debriefing frameworks provide structure to the conversation by outlining phases to the debriefing process that serve specific functions.

- Debriefing approaches are characterized by particular methods of questioning, flow of discussion and overarching goals.

- Debriefing adjuncts, such as the use of video, a co-facilitator or a debriefing script, can help promote discussion and optimize learning outcomes.

- The healthcare simulation community and patients will benefit from determining optimal debriefing methods, defining ideal means of assessing debriefing performance and structuring peer feedback in order to improve learner performance.

Overview

The expansion of simulation-based education (SBE) parallels the equally exciting growth of debriefing in healthcare. Studies provide a growing evidence base that highlights the value of debriefing in SBE and compares variations of debriefing method, structure and content. Skillful and artful debriefing involves thoughtful application of debriefing frameworks, approaches and adjuncts, carefully executed in a manner most likely to promote conversation aligned with learners' needs. We outline various debriefing frameworks, approaches and adjuncts, while providing a toolbox of resources for simulation educators to use during debriefing. We also describe opportunities for debriefing faculty development and highlight key areas for future research to advance the field.

Introduction

Healthcare simulation continues to expand in a wide variety of venues, including undergraduate and post-graduate education as well as continuing professional development. Combined with scenarios designed with clear learning objectives in mind [1], debriefing remains a cornerstone of simulation-based education (SBE). Debriefing refers to the conversation about the simulation experience that traditionally occurs post event (i.e. after the simulation ends) [1]. With debriefing conversations, facilitators strive to promote reflective processes essential for learning [2], but also to provide learners with information about their performance to help them improve [3]. In contrast to debriefing, which is widely viewed as the conversation, feedback refers to the specific information provided to the learner about their performance compared with a defined standard [4]. Recent work has added to our understanding of the alignment between the type of learning objectives and the timing of performance feedback and debriefing conversation [3]. In addition to post-event debriefing strategies, within-event debriefing approaches are gaining traction. Such within-event debriefings, also termed micro-debriefings given their highly focused nature, have shown promise for resuscitation training [5].

Healthcare Simulation Education: Evidence, Theory and Practice, First Edition.
Edited by Debra Nestel, Michelle Kelly, Brian Jolly and Marcus Watson.
© 2018 John Wiley & Sons Ltd. Published 2018 by John Wiley & Sons Ltd.

Conceptually, debriefing provides learners with an important opportunity to reflect on various aspects of the simulation, from concrete events related to what happened to, even more importantly, the rationale for their actions or inactions. Indeed, this reflection represents an essential element of the experiential learning cycle [6]. Once learners have reflected on concrete experiences from the simulation, they work to generalize what they have learnt to generate lessons for future clinical practice [3]. Active experimentation with potential solutions then leads to future experiences, when the experiential learning cycle begins anew. This process of reflection-on-action is the hallmark of SBE and represents an advantage over learning from clinical practice, for which time devoted to deliberate reflection is often a luxury. Thus, debriefing is a conversation in which the reflective process is facilitated by educators [7] or a structured reflection for peer-led debriefings [8]. Meaningful discussion and honest reflection about mistakes and sub-optimal performance are greatly enhanced by a supportive yet challenging learning environment that starts with an effective pre-briefing [9, 10]. While we focus on debriefing in this chapter, educators should recognize that effective SBE also includes a pre-briefing where the learners are orientated to the simulated clinical environment, expectations and roles are clarified, and rules of engagement are explicitly described for the purposes of creating a safe container for learning [9, 10].

The science of debriefing

Is debriefing effective? An extensive meta-analysis conducted across a broad body of research (including non-healthcare fields) reported that organizations can significantly improve the performance of individuals and teams by implementing properly conducted debriefings [11]. A recent systematic review of debriefing in SBE identified 177 studies in which debriefing accompanied an intervention [1]. Debriefing as a component of SBE was associated with improved knowledge, skills and clinical behaviours when compared with no intervention or other forms of instruction. Specific aspects of the debriefing process have been studied as well [1, 12]. A meta-analysis of four studies demonstrated no significant benefit for video-assisted debriefing, while three separate studies of short debriefing combined with

expert modelling demonstrated some benefit when compared with a longer debriefing with no expert modelling of performance [1].

Several additional studies provide further detail regarding some instructional design features of debriefing that may help to enhance learning outcomes. Post-event debriefing has been found to be effective for resuscitation education [13], while within-event debriefing has been effective for endoscopy skills [14]. Student-led debriefing (or self-debriefing) has been effective for certain learner groups [8], and learners prefer debriefing that emphasizes reflection over performance critique [15]. Other researchers have described best practices for debriefing that were developed from an assimilation of existing literature and personal experience [16]. While studies increasingly assess various design elements of debriefing, research comparing one method of debriefing with another is lacking. As a consequence, educators are left to manage the art of debriefing with little guidance on which methods should be used to optimize learning.

The art of debriefing

Healthcare educators can learn the technical skills of debriefing, but *the art of skillful debriefing* involves thoughtful application of a debriefing framework, approaches and adjuncts carefully executed in a manner that is most likely to lead to conversation that addresses the learners' needs.

Debriefing frameworks
A debriefing framework structures the conversation by outlining several phases to the debriefing process that serve specific functions. Various debriefing frameworks have been described in the SBE literature. A commonly applied framework consists of three main phases: the reactions phase (where learner share their visceral emotions and initial reactions to the simulated experience); the analysis phase (where learners engage in reflective discussion and close performance gaps); and the summary phase (where key learning points are highlighted) [17]. Others have advocated for a description phase immediately following the reactions phase, the purpose of which is to have the learners briefly describe their perspective of what the simulation event was about (i.e. clarifying the working diagnosis) [3]. This ensures that

the educator(s) and all learners have a shared mental model regarding the events of the simulation prior to detailed discussion about specific aspects of performance in the analysis phase.

The Gather, Analyze, and Summarize (GAS) framework of debriefing adopted by the American Heart Association [18] also incorporates three phases. In the *Gather* phase the educator invites learners to describe event of the case; the *Analyze* phase has learners reflecting on and analysing their performance, generating ideas for improvement and generalizing discussion points to other contexts; and the *Summarize* phase provides an overview of key take-home messages. Other multiphase frameworks have been described and utilized in SBE. The US Army's after-action review framework includes several distinct phases [19]: define the rules; explain learning objectives; benchmark performance; review expected actions; identify what happened; examine why things happened the way they did; and formalize learning. Lastly, the TeamGAINS approach encourages educators to apply six phases to the debriefing [20]: reactions; discuss the clinical component; transfer from simulation to reality; discussion of behavioural skills; summarization of the learning experience; and supervised practice of clinical skills (if necessary). See Table 21.1.

While many debriefing frameworks exist, little evidence guides their effective use for a given learning context or specific learner groups. However, consistent use of a particular debriefing framework helps educators structure their debriefings and, in turn, may help learners anticipate the flow and nature of conversation once they buy into a particular framework. For novice educators, adopting a debriefing framework can help predictably organize the debriefing process and promotes confidence. More seasoned educators may find that using a debriefing framework helps them to recognize exactly where they are in a debriefing, which can assist with managing time and prioritizing discussion points. The adoption of a particular debriefing framework by a simulation programme can standardize the debriefing process, thus making it easier to provide peer and/or expert feedback on debriefing skills.

Debriefing approaches

Debriefing approaches are characterized by particular methods of questioning, flow of discussion and overarching goals. These include providing information in the form of directive feedback or teaching to knowledge gaps, learner self-assessment, focused facilitation and blending approaches in a single debriefing (Table 21.1) [3, 20]. With directive feedback, the educator aims to identify a performance issue and then provide specific information in order to correct the performance gap [21]. It can be helpful to pair this information with the supportive rationale for corrective behaviours [3]. Directive feedback, while typically unidirectional with information flowing from educator to learner, plays an important role within a debriefing conversation to address specific issues efficiently [4]. Directive feedback and/or teaching is best suited to situations in which knowledge deficits are evident, or if learners are struggling with a particular procedural skill [3].

With learner self-assessment, educators engage learners in a self-reflective process to identify areas of individual or team strengths and weaknesses. The plus-delta method is one form of learner self-assessment where educators ask learners to identify things that went well, and some things that need improvement [3, 7]. This approach to debriefing is educator prompted, but subsequent discussion can be guided by issues or topics generated through learner self-assessment. After learners generate a list of issues, educators can gauge learners' insight based on how they assess their own performance. Aspects of performance that are miscategorized as strengths when they are actually areas of improvement are high-priority items for discussion during the analysis phase of the debriefing.

Educators choose focused facilitation strategies to catalyse discussion that promotes self-reflection, exploration of the underlying reasons for specific behaviours or decisions, identification of solutions to problems and generalization of these solutions to various different contexts. In 'debriefing with good judgement', educators use advocacy inquiry as one form of focused facilitation by pairing a concrete observation from the simulation with their point of view about it, followed by an open-ended question to solicit the learners' perspectives [17, 22]. For example, an educator may notice that during a simulated resuscitation of a child in septic shock, the medication nurse hesitates when the physician orders an incorrect dose of a sedative. Using advocacy inquiry, the educator can probe for the underlying rationale by asking: 'As the team was preparing for intubation, I saw you hesitate when the midazolam was ordered. I was thinking that the midazolam dose

Table 21.1 The art of skilful debriefing: Critical components.

Component of debriefing	Example	Description
Debriefing framework	Debriefing with good judgement	Phases: (1) Reactions; (2) Analysis; (3) Summary
	Promoting Excellence and Reflective Learning in Simulation (PEARLS)	Phases: (1) Reactions; (2) Description; (3) Analysis; (4) Summary
	Gather, Analyze, Summarize	Phases: (1) Gather; (2) Analyze; (3) Summarize
	US Military After-Action Review	Phases: (1) Define the rules; (2) Explain learning objectives; (3) Benchmark performance; (4) Review expected actions; (5) Identify what happened; (6) Examine why things happened the way they did; (7) Formalize learning
	TeamGAINS	Phases: (1) Reactions; (2) Discuss the clinical component; (3) Transfer from simulation to reality; (4) Discussion of behavioural skills; (5) Summarization of the learning experience; (6) Supervised practice of clinical skills (if necessary)
Debriefing Approaches	Providing information	Educators provide specific information to learners in the form of directive feedback or teaching in order to improve future performance
	Learner self-assessment	Educators engage learners in a self-assessment exercise whereby they explore aspects that went well during the simulation, and things that could be improved
	Focused facilitation	The educator facilitates discussion among the learners that encourages self-reflection, exploration of the underlying rationale for specific behaviours/action, identification of solutions to problems and generalization of solutions to various clinical contexts
	Blended approach	The educator thoughtfully and skilfully blends various approaches during a single debriefing. Approaches are carefully selected and adapted based on learner type, learning objectives, learning contexts and time available
Debriefing adjunct	Video debriefing	Video clips are selectively used to highlight aspects of performance during the simulation event
	Co-debriefing	Co-debriefing involves more than one educator contributing to the facilitation process
	Scripted debriefing	Use of a debriefing script or tool helps to standardize the framework and/or approach to debriefing and can serve as a faculty development tool

was high for the child's age, and that perhaps you had noticed that as well. What were your thoughts at that time?' This method uncovers the underlying rationale for a certain behaviour; modifying a learner's rationale for action through discussion and/or teaching is a powerful way to improve future performance. To use advocacy inquiry effectively, educators must be genuinely curious, hold their assumptions loosely and be willing to take the time needed to explore learners' thought processes openly [3].

Guided team self-correction helps learners address their own performance with facilitator support [23]. The educator prompts learners to compare their performance against defined standards of teamwork. Following this, learners are encouraged to analyse and self-correct their behaviours for each component of teamwork. In this sense, guided team self-correction is highly learner centred, but learners must have sufficient prior knowledge and experience to address their own performance deficits adequately. Thus, it is well suited for experienced teams.

Circular questions are a relatively new addition to the healthcare debriefing repertoire [20]. When using circular questions, educators invite someone to reflect on an interaction during the simulation between two other people, thus encouraging a third-person perspective [20]. Sharing insights from this third-person vantage point often triggers discussion that helps uncovers the underlying rationale driving behaviours of interest. This method of questioning also allows individuals and teams to generate solutions to problems uncovered through conversation. Circular questions, in addition to advocacy inquiry and guided team self-correction, play an important role in the TeamGAINS approach to debriefing healthcare teams [20].

Blending approaches to debriefing allows educators to adapt debriefing methods to learner types, learning objectives and learning contexts. No one approach to debriefing is optimal for all intended learning outcomes (e.g. improved clinical reasoning, team working or psychomotor skills). The Promoting Excellence and Augmented Reflective Learning in Simulation (PEARLS) debriefing approach encourages selective blended use of learner self-assessment, focused facilitation strategies and providing information such as directive feedback or targeted teaching during the analysis phase [3]. The PEARLS approach maximizes the strengths of various approaches while striving to minimize weakness, and guides educators as to when each method could be used. Blending debriefing approaches, such as TeamGains [20] or PEARLS [3], require proficiency with each approach to integrate them skilfully and dynamically during a single debriefing.

Debriefing adjuncts

Educators can utilize a number of debriefing adjuncts to maximize the impact of the debriefing experience. Three adjuncts that could be utilized with the debriefing experience include video review, using a co-debriefer and employing a debriefing script. Video-assisted debriefing allows learners and educators to review a relevant clip of the simulation event to prompt further discussion. While a meta-analysis of four video debriefing studies showed equivocal results when compared

to non-video-assisted debriefing [1], the use of video may still demonstrate promise if used in specific situations. Video review can clarify actions and behaviours, illustrate excellent individual or team performance and review unclear communication patterns lost in busy clinical activity [24]. When educators selectively use short video clips and preview for learners what aspects are relevant, this strategy can trigger learner reflection and facilitate meaningful discussion [24].

Co-debriefing involves more than one educator from the same or a different profession facilitating the debriefing conversation together [25]. Effective co-debriefing requires shared understanding of educator roles, debriefing methods and frameworks, learning objectives and a co-debriefing method to leverage the collective experience of all educators. Adding extra educators creates a dynamic between them that should be managed tactfully in a proactive fashion. A co-debriefing checklist encourages open discussion among educators before the simulation session [25]. Educators should meet briefly after each simulation session (e.g. a post-simulation huddle) to discuss positives and negatives from the prior debriefing. If performed consistently and paired with some structure, these huddles represent an important faculty development opportunity that may lead to improved debriefing performance over time.

A debriefing script is a cognitive aid with suggested wording and phrases to guide less experienced educators through the debriefing process. When novice educators use debriefing scripts, learning outcomes for simulation-based paediatric advanced life support training improve [26]. The American Heart Association incorporated debriefing scripts into instructor materials for its advanced life support courses in 2010 to standardize debriefing methods across training programmes [18]. Debriefing scripts also serve as faculty development tools for training new simulation educators [3].

Future directions

The art and science of debriefing have evolved significantly in the past 15 years, primarily devoted to the description of various methods of post-event debriefing. Less attention has been paid to debriefing quality and how to design faculty development opportunities to ensure safe and effective debriefing practice [1, 12].

These aspects represent critical elements for simulation education programme planning related to debriefing and SBE [27].

Debriefing assessment tools

Effective faculty development for debriefing relies on tools that yield valid and reliable information about debriefing quality. Several tools exist that provide both qualitative and quantitative assessments of debriefing practice [28, 29]. Two tools that focus on simulation educator debriefing performance have undergone psychometric testing: the Objective Structured Assessment of Debriefing (OSAD) [28] and the Debriefing Assessment for Simulation in Healthcare (DASH) [29]. The OSAD was developed for debriefing following surgical simulations and for pediatric simulations [30], and demonstrates good inter-rater reliability and internal consistency [28]. It assesses eight core elements using a behaviourally anchored rating scale: approach, learning environment, learner engagement, reaction, reflection, analysis, diagnosis and application [28]. Also a behaviourally anchored rating scale, DASH assesses debriefing across six elements: establishes an engaging learning environment; maintains an engaging learning environment; structures the debriefing in an organized way; provokes engaging discussion; identifies and explores performance gaps; and helps trainees achieve or sustain good future performance [29]. DASH was developed for a variety of specialties and disciplines, and has versions for raters, instructor self-assessment and learner assessment of instructors. The DASH rater (i.e. expert) version demonstrates good evidence of validity and reliability in one limited context. Further generalization of these tools to other learner groups and contexts will aid in the development and ongoing assessment of debriefing skills in simulation educators.

Assessment of debriefing skills for faculty development

Debriefing assessment tools can be used in a formative (or summative) manner to provide objective feedback to educators as part of a debriefing quality assurance programme, where debriefing practice can be measured and tracked over time. Longitudinal data may offer insights into retention and decay of debriefing skills, and may highlight specific faculty development needs for individual educators [27]. How best to provide feedback on debriefing performance for both novice and experienced debriefers is poorly understood.

Peer feedback is a potential means to enhance the feedback culture surrounding debriefing within simulation programmes. Peer observation and feedback have already been shown to be an effective means of improving clinical teaching [31]. Application of peer observation and feedback for debriefing skills would likely yield similar results. However, simulation educators need guidance on how to provide honest and constructive peer feedback through faculty development that allows for deliberate practice in facilitating feedback conversations on debriefing performance [27].

Debriefing research

Finally, progress in debriefing assessment and faculty development lies in well-designed research that augments our understanding of how these advances can affect learners' educational outcomes. Important areas for future research include the various factors that influence debriefing (e.g. timing, length, structure); how adjuncts can further enhance debriefing (e.g. video, scripting, multiple facilitators); comparative effectiveness research on debriefing methods and their impact on educational and clinical outcomes; and characteristics of faculty development in debriefing (e.g. frequency, timing, content and structure) that benefit both educators and ultimately learners [32]. Researchers should carefully isolate the independent variable and ensure that all simulation-specific confounders are carefully controlled for in the study design [32, 33].

Conclusion

Debriefing is a critical and rapidly evolving part of SBE. The application of frameworks, structured approaches and debriefing adjuncts provides educators with a toolbox of resources that promotes learning from SBE. Future debriefing research should define optimal methods and identify strategies to enhance debriefing skills through faculty development.

References

1 Cheng, A., Eppich, W., Grant, V. *et al.* (2014) Debriefing for technology-enhanced simulation: a systematic review and meta-analysis. *Med Educ*, **48** (7), 657–66.

2 Kihlgren, P., Spanager, L. and Dieckmann, P. (2014) Investigating novice doctors' reflections in debriefings after simulation scenarios. *Med Teach.*, **5**, 1–7.

3 Eppich, W. and Cheng, A. (2015) Promoting Excellence and Reflective Learning in Simulation (PEARLS): development and rationale for a blended approach to health care simulation debriefing. *Simul Healthc*, **10** (2), 106–15.

4 van de Ridder, J.M., Stokking, K.M., McGaghie, W.C. and ten Cate, O.T. (2008) What is feedback in clinical education? *Med Educ*, **42** (2), 189–97.

5 Eppich, W., Hunt, E.A., Duval-Arnauld, J. *et al.* (2015) Structuring feedback and debriefing to achieve mastery learning goals. *Acad Med*, **90** (11), 1501–8.

6 Kolb, D. (1984) *Experiential learning: experience as a source of learning and development*, Upper Saddle River, NJ, Prentice Hall.

7 Fanning, R.M. and Gaba, D.M. (2007) The role of debriefing in simulation-based learning. *Simul Healthc*, **2** (2), 115–25.

8 Boet, S., Bould, M.D., Sharma, B. *et al.* (2013) Within-team debriefing versus instructor-led debriefing for simulation-based education: a randomized controlled trial. *Ann Surg*, **258** (1), 53–8.

9 Kolbe, M., Grande, B. and Spahn, D.R. (2015) Briefing and debriefing during simulation-based training and beyond: content, structure, attitude and setting. *Best Pract Res Clin Anaesthesiol*, **29** (1), 87–96.

10 Rudolph, J.W., Raemer, D.B. and Simon, R. (2014) Establishing a safe container for learning in simulation: the role of presimulation briefing. *Simul Healthc*, **9** (6), 339–49.

11 Tannenbaum, S.I. and Cerasoli, C.P. (2013) Do team and individual debriefs enhance performance? *A meta-analysis. Hum Factors.*, **55**, 231–45.

12 Garden, A.L., Le Fevre, D.M., Waddington, H.L. and Weller, J.M. (2015) Debriefing after simulation-based non-technical skill training in healthcare: a systematic review. *Anaesth Intensive Care.*, **43**, 300–8.

13 Van Heukelom, J.N., Begaz, T. and Treat, R. (2010) Comparison of post-simulation debriefing versus in-simulation debriefing in medical simulation. *Simul Healthc.*, **5**, 91–7.

14 Walsh, C.M., Ling, S.C., Wang, C.S. and Carnahan, H. (2009) Concurrent versus terminal feedback: it may be better to wait. *Acad Med*, **84** (Suppl), 54–7.

15 Dreifuerst, K.T. (2012) Using debriefing for meaningful learning to foster development of clinical reasoning in simulation. *J Nurs Educ*, **51**, 326–33.

16 Lyons, R., Lazzara, E.H., Benishek, L.E. *et al.* (2015) Enhancing the effectiveness of team debriefings in medical simulation: more best practices. *Jt Comm J Qual Patient Saf*, **41** (3), 115–25.

17 Rudolph, J., Simon, R., Dufresne, R. and Raemer, D. (2006) There's no such thing as "nonjudgmental" debriefing: a theory and method for debriefing with good judgment. *Sim Healthc*, **1** (1), 49–55.

18 Cheng, A., Rodgers, D., Van Der Jagt, E. *et al.* (2012) Evolution of the pediatric advanced life support course: enhanced learning with a new debriefing tool and web-based module for pediatric advanced life support instructors. *Ped Crit Care Med*, **13** (5), 589–95.

19 Sawyer, T. and Deering, S. (2013) Adaptation of the U.S. Army's After-Action Review (AAR) to simulation debriefing in healthcare. *Sim Healthc*, **8** (6), 388–97.

20 Kolbe, M., Weiss, M., Grote, G. *et al.* (2013) TeamGAINS: a tool for structured debriefings for simulation-based team trainings. *BMJ Qual Saf*, **22** (7), 541–53.

21 Archer, J.C. (2010) State of the science in health professional education: effective feedback. *Med Educ*, **44** (1), 101–8.

22 Rudolph, J.W., Simon, R., Raemer, D.B. and Eppich, W.J. (2008) Debriefing as formative assessment: closing performance gaps in medical education. *Acad Emerg Med*, **15** (11), 1010–16.

23 Smith-Jentsch, K.A., Cannon-Bowers, J.A., Tannenbaum, S.I. and Salas, E. (2008) Guided team self-correction: impacts on team mental models, processes, and effectiveness. *Small Gr Res*, **39** (3), 303–27.

24 Krogh, K., Bearman, M. and Nestel, D. (2015) Expert practice of video-assisted debriefing: an Australian qualitative study. *Clin Simul Nurs.*, **11**, 180–87.

25 Cheng, A., Palaganas, J., Rudolph, J. *et al.* (2015) Co-debriefing for simulation-based education: a primer for facilitators. *Simul Healthc.*, **10**, 69–75.

26 Cheng, A., Hunt, E., Donoghue, A. *et al.* (2013) Examining pediatric resuscitation education using simulation and scripted debriefing: a multicenter randomized trial. *JAMA Pediatr*, **167** (6), 528–36.

27 Cheng, A., Grant, V., Dieckmann, P. *et al.* (2015) Faculty development for simulation programs: five issues for the future of debriefing training. *Simul Healthc*, **10** (4), 217–22.

28 Arora, S., Ahmed, M., Paige, J. *et al.* (2012) Objective structured assessment of debriefing (OSAD): bringing science to the art of debriefing in surgery. *Ann Surg*, **256** (6), 982–8.

29 Brett-Fleegler, M., Rudolph, J., Eppich, W. *et al.* (2012) Debriefing assessment for simulation in healthcare: development and psychometric properties. *Simul Healthc*, **7** (5), 288–94.

30 Runnacles, J., Thomas, L., Sevdalis, N. *et al.* (2014) Development of a tool to improve performance debriefing and learning: the paediatric objective structured assessment of debriefing (OSAD) tool. *Postgrad Med J*, **90** (1069), 613–21.

31 Steinert, Y., Mann, K., Centeno, A. *et al.* (2006) A systematic review of faculty development initiatives designed to improve teaching effectiveness in medical education: BEME Guide No. 8. *Med Teach*, **28**, 497–526.

32 Raemer, D., Anderson, M., Cheng, A. *et al.* (2011) Research regarding debriefing as part of the learning process. *Simul Healthc.*, **6**, s52–s57.

33 Cheng, A., Kessler, D., MacKinnon, R., *et al.* (2016) Reporting Guidelines for Health Care Simulation Research: Extensions for the CONSORT and STROBE Statements. *Simulation in Healthcare.* **11** (4):238–248.

SECTION V
Innovations in healthcare simulation practice

CHAPTER 22

Simulation of home births: Developing safe practices

Arunaz Kumar & Debra Nestel

KEY MESSAGES

- The safety of a home birth programme can be strengthened through an in-situ simulation workshop.

- A real-life emergency simulation in real time can not only provide participants with an opportunity to practise clinical skills in preparation for rare clinical emergencies, but also enable them to improve their communication and team-working capabilities.

Overview

Birth at home is a safe and appropriate choice for healthy women with a low-risk pregnancy. However, it carries a small risk of a birth emergency requiring immediate, skilled management to optimize maternal and/or neonatal outcomes [1]. We developed a simulation-based education workshop designed to run in a home-based setting to assist with emergency training for midwives undertaking home birth care, and present an evaluation of that workshop by assessing participants' satisfaction and their response regarding key learning issues. Both midwifery and paramedical staff were invited to participate in an in-situ simulation workshop (in a community home), where the teams were presented with simulated emergency clinical scenarios, which needed to be managed in real time. This was found to be a useful tool by staff who participate in home birth or intrapartum patient transfer. Developing clear communication and team work were found to be the most important learning messages from the activity.

What was the need?

Birth either at a hospital or at home may rarely present with sudden and unforeseen complications that require the attending healthcare providers to manage these situations in a timely manner and with effective teamwork [2]. Teaching these skills to healthcare professionals is a challenge, as some of these emergencies, like shoulder dystocia, postpartum haemorrhage and neonatal respiratory distress, are uncommon, hence resulting in a poor clinical exposure for the attending staff members, especially in a low-risk setting. Simulation-based educational workshops have been integrated into hospital-based credentialling programmes to upskill staff members with management skills and emergency clinical procedures, and also to equip them with team-working skills to enable them to manage these obstetric emergency situations safely.

Although simulation-based educational programmes provide training for hospital-based emergencies, similar programmes have so far not been introduced to manage the complications of a home birth. However, with the improvement in healthcare facilities, and the availability of more birth choices for women, there appears to have been a recent increase in interest in home births, hence unmasking the need for the development of simulation programmes that can support the learning requirements of the staff attending births at home.

Birth simulation programmes have typically focused on teaching clinical or procedural skills and/or on team work. An example of such a training model is the Practical Obstetric Multi-Professional Training (PROMPT) model [3], where multidisciplinary teams involved in

Healthcare Simulation Education: Evidence, Theory and Practice, First Edition.
Edited by Debra Nestel, Michelle Kelly, Brian Jolly and Marcus Watson.

maternity care learn together to manage a simulated emergency on a birth unit as a team. The PROMPT model of teaching was developed in the UK and has successfully demonstrated improved skills in team work and patient management, leading to better clinical outcomes [4]. In a hospital-based setting, this involves midwives, obstetric, anaesthetic and paediatric clinical staff working together through an obstetric simulated emergency in real time.

What did we do?

Based on the concept of the PROMPT model, we have introduced a home birth–based model with an in-situ simulation conducted in a home-based setting. The workshop was introduced to improve the performance of participants (midwifery or paramedical staff) in managing these complications safely and efficiently. The participants' response to the home birth simulation workshop was evaluated to explore the key learning achieved through this activity.

Method

As part of accreditation, the Practical Obstetric Multi-Professional Training workshop is undertaken annually by all staff, as an 'in-house' training session at the hospital maternity unit. Obstetricians, anaesthetists, paediatricians and midwives train together as a team, with a focus on all facets of clinical practice (including team work and communication), where the participants encounter a simulated obstetric or neonatal emergency and are later given group feedback on their performance. Adapted from the successful Practical Obstetric Multi-Professional Training (PROMPT) workshop, we designed an in-situ home birth workshop to upskill midwives involved in running this particular service.

Workshop details
Setting
The home-based PROMPT workshop was designed for training for home birth, with its focus on working within the scope of practice of the home birth staff and managing situations with limited resources to provide safe care in a home-based setting.

To enhance the fidelity (or realism) of the simulation, the workshop was delivered in a community home (in-situ). The equipment used for training was the home birth kit used by midwives in a real home birth. Replicating real home birth practice, only two midwives (occasionally accompanied by the paramedical staff) were active participants in each scenario of this programme.

Simulated emergency scenarios
The workshop covered five clinical emergency scenarios, which would start with a phone call where a woman in (simulated) labour would make a telephone call to the home birth midwife. Following the initial encounter, the scenario unfolded with the occurrence of intrapartum, postpartum or neonatal complications. At the start of each scenario, a different pair of midwives and paramedics were recruited to participate without prior knowledge of what was about to occur in scenario, and the rest of the participants were silent observers in the scenario.

The task required participants to identify and manage the emergency with stabilization of the mother or baby in real time, using the equipment provided in the home birth kit. The simulation usually required participants to make a phone call to the birth unit, obstetricians and to the Emergency Services Telecommunication Authority (ESTA) by initiating a mock phone call (arranged beforehand with the emergency services). The ESTA staff responded to the situation by handling the distress phone call. The MICA paramedic staff then joined the scenario and, together with the home birth midwives, managed the situation as a team, during which they were required to use the woman's partner's help where considered appropriate and to communicate frequently with the in-hospital staff, including the midwife in charge of the birth unit and the obstetrician on call. Most scenarios culminated with the transfer of the mother and/or baby to hospital in the ambulance.

Eight to twelve midwives and two to four paramedical staff participated in each simulation session, which lasted half a day. In most scenarios, hybrid simulation was used, where the simulated 'patient' was incorporated with a birthing model (Model-med International Pty Ltd, Melbourne, Australia) for pelvic examination, birth and internal manoeuvres. The role of the simulated patient was played by one of the trained home birth midwives, with detailed instructions provided to

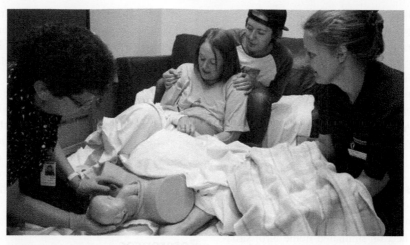

Figure 22.1 Hybrid simulation incorporating a woman with a task trainer to replicate a birthing scenario authentically.

her by the PROMPT educator to portray a woman in labour (see Figure 22.1). Scenarios involving newborn resuscitation used a SimBaby newborn model (Laerdal Medical, Norway).

Each scenario was followed by a debriefing session involving all participants, where they were encouraged to reflect on their performance and discuss their challenges and views with the other participants regarding how the experience of the simulation would influence their clinical practice. Debriefing included feedback given to the participants by an experienced PROMPT midwifery educator about their performance in the simulation, which took approximately 30 minutes for each scenario. There was an opportunity for participants to relate to their clinical experiences and obtain peer feedback on ways to improve their performance.

What was the impact?

Both midwifery and paramedical staff found the simulation scenarios and the debriefing helpful. The most frequently cited learning was related to the communication skills of the home birth midwife, such as face-to-face communication (to the other midwife, MICA paramedical staff or the woman's partner) and by telephone to ESTA, the obstetrician on call and the hospital midwife in charge. The focus was on clarity, such as communicating precisely and concisely during handovers to paramedics and timely and accurate documentation.

The second most important learning was related to 'being prepared', which included both anticipation of the problem and preparation of equipment required to manage the situation. The importance of identifying how the home birth care environment influenced the outcome was recognized, which included familiarization with protocols, attending to the environment for safety of the baby and mother and transport arrangements, such as requesting two ambulances.

Participants identified safety as underpinning much of the learning, for instance on using all available resources, including asking for the partner to help. Team work and insight into others' roles were identified as key learning objectives.

Finally, the role of realism in the simulation was highlighted. People were interacting with others in their usual 'real' roles (colleagues from midwifery, paramedical staff and obstetrics), the simulation took place in a real home, activities were undertaken in real time, and the scenario challenges were realistic and the psychosocial fidelity believable. The staff members engaged well with the activity and thought that the simulation was useful to support their practice by providing 'learning in a non-threatening environment'. The debriefing was perceived to provide reflection on the team's performance in the scenario, with a view to positively influencing team attitudes and behaviours in the future. The debriefing also provided a forum for participants to discuss how they will prognosticate, prioritize and strategize their course of action in the most efficient way.

The positive impact of this activity on participants' learning encouraged the health service to amalgamate this exercise as part of an annual credentialling requirement for all home birth midwives working within the health service. This simulation-based teaching, complemented by the annual completion of the hospital-based PROMPT workshop, has assisted home birth midwives to maintain the upskilling required to face those rare clinical emergency situations.

What lessons were learnt?

The intervention was beneficial in enabling participants to practise and reflect on simulated home birth situations, which were similar to real clinical challenges. The participants could compare and self-assess their technical skills, but, more importantly, recognized the value in the opportunity to communicate effectively with colleagues and with the support person at home, and to be prepared with a back-up plan if complications occurred.

The development of a relationship for working together is an investment requiring time and effort, and activities such as these help to improve a team-building approach towards facing common challenges. The exchange of information under relatively stressful simulated situations helped in identifying and acknowledging the mutual support that teams provide each other. The 'handover and overlap of management with the ambulance staff' provided a sharing of clinical information with a focus on patient safety at all times. This was considered important, since most home birth complications require an expeditious transfer to hospital for further observation, even after the required management plan has been enacted [5].

Both structural fidelity (how the simulator appears) and functional fidelity (what a simulator does) contribute to the success of a simulation programme [6]. The value of using a functional and instructional design that resembles the clinical tasks cannot be understated, and this workshop strengthens this viewpoint. Of note is the concept of *in-situ simulation* (the salient feature of this workshop), which has been shown to contribute to both physical (due to the context and the location) and psychological fidelity (due to realism perceived by the participants) [6]. Hence, in-situ simulation is described as 'a team-based simulation strategy that occurs on the actual patient care units involving actual healthcare team members within their own working environment' [7].

The learning acquired through the simulation has since then also been put to the test when home birth teams have encountered challenging clinical situations similar to the simulated scenarios and were able to relate them directly to the simulation experience. The impact on change in clinical practice and outcome is under study at the time of this publication and remains to be reported.

References

1 National Institute for Health and Care Excellence. Intrapartum care for healthy women and babies. December 2014 [cited 15 September 2016]. Available at: https://www.nice.org.uk/guidance/CG190

2 Catling-Paul, C., Coddington, R.L., Foureur, M.J. and Homer, C.S.E. (2013) on behalf of the Birthplace in Australia Study and the National Publicly-funded Homebirth Consortium. Publicly funded homebirth in Australia: a review of maternal and neonatal outcomes over 6 years. *Med J Aust*, **198**, 616–20.

3 Crofts, J.F., Ellis, D., Draycott, T.J. *et al.* (2007) Change in knowledge of midwives and obstetricians following obstetric emergency training: a randomised controlled trial of local hospital, simulation centre and teamwork training. *BJOG*, **114** (12), 1534–41.

4 Shoushtarian, M., Barnett, M., McMahon, F. and Ferris, J. (2014) Impact of introducing Practical Obstetric Multi-Professional Training (PROMPT) into maternity units in Victoria. *Australia. BJOG Int J Obstet Gynaecol.*, **121** (13), 1710–18.

5 Blix, E., Kumle, M., Kjærgaard, H. *et al.* (2014) Transfer to hospital in planned home births: a systematic review. *BMC Pregnancy Childbirth.*, **14**, 179. doi: 10.1186/1471-2393-14-179

6 Hamstra, S.J., Brydges, R., Hatala, R. *et al.* (2014) Reconsidering fidelity in simulation-based training. *Acad Med*, **89** (3), 387–92.

7 Sørensen, J.L., Van der Vleuten, C., Lindschou, J. *et al.* (2013) 'In situ simulation' versus 'off site simulation' in obstetric emergencies and their effect on knowledge, safety attitudes, team performance, stress, and motivation: study protocol for a randomized controlled trial. *Trials.*, **14**, 220. doi: 10.1186/1745-6215-14-220

CHAPTER 23

Optimizing learning in simulation-based education using video-reflexivity

Suzanne Gough

KEY MESSAGES

- Video-reflexive methods are becoming increasingly popular in healthcare to improve educational outcomes, healthcare practice and patient safety.
- Video-reflexivity illustrates the complex interconnectivity of participants and the simulated learning environment.
- Video-reflexivity findings have influenced curriculum development and delivery as well as improvements in the design of new simulation facilities.

Overview

This case study provides a brief overview of how the combination of simulation-based education (SBE) and video-reflexivity can be successfully used to optimize learning opportunities for healthcare students. This chapter presents the context, methods and impact on students' learning and changes to the curriculum and simulated learning environment (SLE) facilities. Potential opportunities afforded when combining SBE and video-reflexivity are highlighted from findings of a sequential explanatory mixed-methods doctoral study, in which undergraduate physiotherapists took part in the assessment of a deteriorating respiratory patient. Considerations are proposed for other educational programmes wishing to embed elements of video-reflexivity within SBE.

What was the need?

Healthcare educators have a responsibility to promote student engagement and facilitate students' professional development during their studies. Central to this is fostering the students' progression as autonomous practitioners who can review their own learning in order to facilitate understanding and propose developments in their own practice, particularly in relation to professional knowledge, skills, attitudes and behaviours [1].

Video-reflexivity has been described as a process whereby participants replay ethnographic video footage for review and discussion [2]. The combination of video-ethnography and video-reflexive methods (known as video-reflexive ethnography, VRE) is becoming increasingly popular in healthcare research [2, 3]. VRE has also been used by researchers in the quest to improve patient safety in healthcare [2, 3]. To the author's knowledge, no previous studies had explored the personal experiences or errors encountered within the simulated learning environment (SLE) using VRE. There is also limited evidence of how digital technologies have been employed to support learning or reflexive practice within physiotherapy.

What did we do?

This case study reports findings from phase two of a sequential mixed-methods design [4]. The research was based on the perspectives of multiplicity and complexity, drawing on the social constructivism view that knowledge and meaning are constructed, developed and communicated through interactions between humans and their world [5]. This was aligned with an interpretative approach using VRE methodology [2, 3].

Healthcare Simulation Education: Evidence, Theory and Practice, First Edition.
Edited by Debra Nestel, Michelle Kelly, Brian Jolly and Marcus Watson.
© 2018 John Wiley & Sons Ltd. Published 2018 by John Wiley & Sons Ltd.

The research approach used video-observation and focused, unedited video-reflexive interviews. These methods were selected to capture multiple perspectives (approaches and understandings) of the complexity of managing a deteriorating simulated patient (SP). Roskell and Cross described the complex interactions that a respiratory physiotherapist undertakes to function effectively within their clinical environment, including constant observation of the patient, monitors and equipment located within the visual field around the patient's bed space or, in this case, the simulated side ward [6]. The importance of the physiotherapist's need to maintain situational awareness to function efficiently while optimally managing the patient, and filtering unwanted stimuli from the environment, was also recognized [6]. With this in mind, the study needed to be able to illuminate these concurrent phenomena, including the differences between participants in their interactions and abilities. It would not be possible to maintain the essential and embedded features of these phenomena if they were solely measured and reduced to the testing of generated hypotheses.

This case study draws on findings from two of the research questions:

- To what extent are final-year physiotherapy students able independently to manage a deteriorating simulated cardiorespiratory patient?
- To what extent are final-year physiotherapy students able independently to recognize errors within a simulated scenario?

Methods

Twenty-one final-year pre-registration (BSc Hons) physiotherapy students were invited to participate in a simulation scenario and video-reflexive interview. They took part in an immersive authentic simulation scenario designed to replicate the complexity of an emergency on-call physiotherapy situation. The scenario required the students to undertake an assessment and provide appropriate management of an acutely deteriorating patient. Two specific methods of promoting reflexivity were utilized:

- Video-recording the participants in the simulation scenario,
- Participants being able immediately to review their respective unedited simulation scenario video.

The respective participants' video was displayed on a 21″ Apple iMac (which enabled large-screen viewing).

QuickTime computer software was used to capture the screen and audio of the interview as one movie file. The students reviewed their respective unedited simulation videos during the video-reflexive interview. The interview consisted of 21 questions that aimed to promote self-reflection, while engaging in a critical discussion of themselves and their cultural (clinical) practices [7]. The interview questions were specifically designed to reflect the research questions.

All 12 simulation and interview videos were transcribed verbatim, then analysed using video-analysis software (Studiocode, http://www.studiocodegroup.com/) and a thematic framework approach [8].

What was the impact?

The use of VRE in this study illuminated the multilayered impact of personal experiences, ethics and behaviours on their practices, clinical reasoning, clinical decisions, dynamics and the complexities and interconnectivity of participants to the SLE [2, 3, 7, 9]. The findings of this study have demonstrated that the combination of SBE and video-reflexivity has the potential to optimize learning and enhance both professional practice, patient safety [2, 7] and organizational change. Additional benefits of using video-reflexivity included the potential to provide an in-depth exploration of 'learning' and the impact of objects and artefacts embodied within the scenario and SLE, by drawing on the theories of *complexity* and *cultural-historical activity* [7, 9]. Summaries of both learner and organizational impact are now presented.

Learner impact

Video observation identified similarities and differences in patient assessment and management approaches. The students' assessment approaches were generally unstructured, despite students trying to use a standardized assessment and management approach. Management approaches also varied in relation to a specific intervention, order and timing of events/actions. During the video-reflexive interview, students explored the content of their respective simulation videos, attempting to make sense of the occurrence and highlighting the impact of personal experiences, which they perceived may have been central to their actions, clinical decisions and the cause or mitigation of errors in their practice. The students demonstrated a capacity for openness and observation, working within the uncertainty and complexity of a deteriorating scenario and offering known or alternative solutions. They demonstrated mindfulness as they vocalized being aware of themselves, demonstrating a shared interest in what they and others did. Students also questioned their own knowledge, technical and non-technical skills (strengths and deficits), professionalism, errors encountered and realism of the simulated experience in a manner that had an impact on themselves and how they related to the patient and each other within the SLE [2, 3, 9]. The impact of academic, clinical placement and personal experiences was highlighted as positive influential factors on their subject knowledge (physiotherapy management of a deteriorating patient), skill acquisition and behaviours. Students also reflected on the lack of respiratory-related placements or practical opportunities (e g suctioning or moving and handling patients) and limited experience of immersive scenarios, which may have negatively affected their ability to manage the simulated patient.

Organizational impact

The findings of this study have already influenced several aspects of curriculum development and delivery as well as improvements in the usage of the university's new SLE facilities. An 'integrated simulation-based education framework' was developed from the literature, theoretical and methodological approaches and findings of this study [4]. Implementation of this framework has led to improvements in scenario design, formalizing debriefing practices and ensuring that linked learning activities are overtly articulated to students. Findings from the video analysis and VRE interviews have influenced scenario design in relation to fostering:

- *Emergence*: acknowledging diverse ways of thinking, acting and being responsive to change.
- *Materiality*: consideration of the effects of equipment and the environment.
- *Attunement*: providing opportunities to enhance non-technical skills such as situational awareness in order to sense what is unfolding.
- *Disturbance*: introducing interruptions to routine practices.
- *Experimentation*: providing diverse learning and feedback opportunities [9].

The identification of errors encountered in the simulation scenario also led to a series of curriculum and SLE design changes. The emphasis of human factors and their effect on patient safety has been made more explicit in simulation scenarios and debriefing activities, and additional learning resources have been created. The study identified a gap between learning and the actual practice of knowledge and skills gained from the physiotherapy curriculum, in particular relating to knowledge and skill deficits (*error-producing factors*) [10]. The provision of additional 'flipped classroom' [11] resources (educational videos and podcasts) has been introduced to support repetitive practice of essential technical and non-technical skills required to manage cardiorespiratory and acutely deteriorating patients. Multiple policies around oxygen therapy (a *latent error*) have been replaced with a single guideline to minimize confusion and error [10]. The combination of a lack of hand-washing facilities (an *error-producing factor*) in the previous SLE and identification of infection control and moving and handling violations (*active failures*) [10] have also contributed to the design of the new SLE facilities at the university.

What lessons were learnt?

This study highlighted the power of video-reflexivity to explore and uncover the multiple and complex realities of managing a deteriorating simulated patient, which are constructed via social, verbal and non-verbal interactions with the patient, others and the environment [2, 9]. The visualization and narratives provided by students during the video-reflexive interview offered the ability to understand the complexity of learning within the SLE. Carefully planned and executed simulation scenarios and video-reflexive methods can offer a safe learning environment to allow students to explore routine, evolving and complex situations while enabling them to learn to be become comfortable with making and exploring errors (mistakes/violations).

Table 23.1 highlights the potential opportunities afforded when combining SBE and video-reflexive methods, drawing on interactions identified in this study, and poses considerations for other educational programmes. This study highlighted the benefits of exploring the dimensions of learning beyond metrics to make sense of the dynamics within the simulated

Table 23.1 Interactions and considerations for educational programmes when using simulation and video-reflexive methods.

Interactions identified through simulation and video-reflexivity	Considerations for educational programmes
Multiple complexities of learning within the simulated environment • Video reflexivity illustrated the multilayered impact of personal experiences, codes of practice, conformity/non-conformity, errors, dynamics and the complexities of interconnectivity of students and the SLE.	• SBE design requires complex thought and preparation to construct optimal learning experiences carefully. Drawing on learning (adult, social and cognitive) theories and educational practices aligned to SBE may help to optimize learning. • The identification of routine/non-routine actions, relevant codes of professional practice, conformity and creativity highlights the need to increase the focus on different types of thinking when designing and debriefing scenarios. • Simulation provides opportunities for students to take managed risks in a safe learning environment. However, such risks and potential/actual errors should be appropriately discussed during the debriefing (feedback). • Socio-material theories (complexity and cultural-historical activity) are highly relevant to scenario and SLE design considerations [9]. For example, complexity theory raises key considerations for scenario and SLE design in relation to the effects of *emergence* (diverse ways of thinking, acting and being responsive to change), *materiality* (equipment and environment), *attunement* (listening and touching to sense what is unfolding), *disturbance* (fostering/amplifying the disturbance of routine practices) and *experimentation* (providing multiple, diverse learning and feedback opportunities) [9].
Collective competency and enhanced intelligence • Students interact to manage a deteriorating patient, communicating decisions to reach a shared level of understanding (collective competency) and exploring how they enacted the process of knowing together (enhanced intelligence).	• Video-reflexive methods and facilitator-led debriefing strategies can be used to explore the development of collective competence and enhanced intelligence, which may help to understand how these skills can be translated to healthcare practice. • Facilitating opportunities to explore the process of 'knowing' for and alongside each other potentially equips students to engage with complexity, influence professionalism and have an impact on patient safety [3].
Learner insight • Students lacked insight into some errors encountered during the scenario, predominantly relating to knowledge and skills (relating to physiotherapy assessment components, intervention and moving and handling/infection control violations).	• The use of simulation and video-reflexive methods provides potential opportunities for facilitators to identify students who lack insight into their own knowledge, skills, attitudes and behaviours. A structured facilitator-led debriefing can provide an opportunity to regain balanced discussion between achievements, creativity, the need to appreciate professional boundaries, codes of conduct, policies and procedures, while raising learners' awareness of deficits in knowledge, skills, attitudes and desired behaviours. Consideration of further remediation opportunities may be required.

environment. This study highlights that as educationalists, we need to be mindful that learning is highly complex, always contextual and continually evolving through social interaction [9]. It is essential therefore that evaluation can reflect this multiplicity. Pragmatic measures are suitable for technical and non-technical skills, but the emergence of new holistic evaluation methods, which draw on both qualitative and quantitative approaches, may have a place in helping to establish the extent to which transformations in learning and/or patient care are realized, or not, by the learner [12]. Such approaches offer greater enlightenment on the links between educational interventions and outcomes. By employing and triangulating qualitative and quantitative approaches to consider multiple levels of impact, the complexities of learning can be explored, identifying areas of best practice and helping to remedy any deficits, to enhance the transformation between theory and practice [12].

References

1 Chartered Society of Physiotherapy (2013) *Physiotherapy framework: putting physiotherapy behaviours, values, knowledge and skills into practice*, Chartered Society of Physiotherapy, London.

2 Carroll, K. (2009) Outsider, insider, alongside: examining reflexivity in hospital–based video research. *Int J Mult Res Approach*, **3** (3), 246–63.

3 Iedema, R. (2011) Creating safety by strengthening clinicians' capacity for reflexivity. *BMJ Qual Saf*, **20** (Suppl 1), i83–i86.

4 Gough, S. (2016) *The use of simulation based education in cardio-respiratory physiotherapy. Unpublished doctoral thesis*, Manchester Metropolitan University, Manchester.

5 Crotty, M. (1998) *The foundations of social research: meaning and perspective in the research process*, Sydney, Allen and Unwin.

6 Roskell, C. and Cross, V. (1998) Attention limitation and learning in physiotherapy. *Physiotherapy*, **84** (3), 118–25.

7 Iedema, R., Mesman, J. and Carroll, K. (2013) Does the complexity of care call for 'research complexity'? in *Visualising health care practice improvement: innovation from within* (eds R. Iedema, J. Mesman and K. Carroll), Radcliffe, London, pp. 41–66.

8 Ritchie, J. and Spencer, L. (1994) Analyzing qualitative data, in *Qualitative data analysis for applied policy research* (eds A. Bryman and R.G. Burgess), Routledge, London, pp. 173–94.

9 Fenwick, T. and Dahlgren, M.A. (2015) Towards socio-material approaches in simulation-based education: lessons from complexity theory. *Med Educ*, **49** (4), 359–67.

10 Reason, J.T. (1999) *Human error*, Cambridge University Press, New York, Cambridge.

11 Roehl, A., Reddy, S.L. and Shannon, G.J. (2013) The flipped classroom: an opportunity to engage millennial students through active learning strategies. *J Fam Consum Sci*, **105** (2), 44–9.

12 Drescher, U., Warren, F. and Norton, K. (2004) Towards evidence-based practice in medical training: making evaluations more meaningful. *Med Educ*, **38** (12), 1288–94.

Further Reading

1 Fenwick, T. and Nerland, M. (2011) *Reconceptualising professional learning*, Routledge, London.

2 Iedema, R., Mesman, J. and Carroll, K. (eds) (2013) *Visualising health care practice improvement: innovation from within*, Radcliffe, London.

CHAPTER 24

Conversations about organ and tissue donation: The role of simulation

Jonathan Gatward, Leigh McKay & Michelle Kelly

KEY MESSAGES

- The complex issue of organ and tissue donation (OTD) is discussed with families of dead or dying patients in times of acute grief and distress, making these conversations especially challenging.
- Simulation-based education using professional actors and a thorough debriefing process can provide clinicians with valuable practice and reflection, resulting in increased knowledge, self-awareness and confidence.

Overview

A simulation-based education programme was created to help clinicians in New South Wales (NSW) lead difficult conversations about organ and tissue donation (OTD) with the families of dead or dying patients. Participants led a planning meeting with the Intensive Care Unit (ICU) team, then a family donation conversation (FDC) with the family of the potential donor. Professional actors played family members during scenarios based on real cases. A three-stage debriefing process including video-reflexive feedback followed the FDC. Eighty participants completed the training, which was universally well received, with participants reporting a wide range of educational benefits and increased confidence. There has been an increase in the family consent rate for OTD in NSW over the duration of the programme. Whether the training contributed to this increase is unclear at this stage.

What was the need?

Organ and tissue transplantation is an effective treatment for people with end-stage disease [1]. Unfortunately, donation rates in Australia have failed to increase in line with the growth of the population in recent years [1].

An important influence on the number of donors is family consent. Legally and ethically, organ and tissue donation (OTD) is dependent on informed decision making and consent by the donor family. It is common practice in Australia for the managing intensive care unit (ICU) doctor to lead the family donation conversation (FDC). These conversations can be extremely difficult, irrespective of the clinician's level of expertise or experience. The family is often emotionally and physically overwhelmed by the circumstances, which are frequently sudden and unexpected. This can influence their ability to understand and process the complex medical information required to make informed decisions, including about OTD. For several years in New South Wales (NSW), the rate of family consent for OTD has been around 50%, which is well below the national target of 75% [2]. Reasons for this are unclear.

Traditionally, clinicians have received little formal training in communication skills and can be poorly prepared to understand acute grief reactions. They may also have a lack of knowledge about the OTD process. Opportunities to rehearse and reflect on FDCs are scarce, resulting in clinicians developing their approach either from observing colleagues or by trial and error.

Healthcare Simulation Education: Evidence, Theory and Practice, First Edition.
Edited by Debra Nestel, Michelle Kelly, Brian Jolly and Marcus Watson.
© 2018 John Wiley & Sons Ltd. Published 2018 by John Wiley & Sons Ltd.

The Australian Organ and Tissue Authority was established in 2009 to implement a national reform package [1]. One of the strategic priorities of the reform was to increase consent rates for OTD by delivering specialized education to organ donation specialists. A professional education package (PEP) was developed to provide training in conducting FDCs and supporting families to make a proactive, informed and enduring decision [3]. In NSW a group of clinicians who had completed the PEP became 'designated requesters' (DRs): ICU doctors, donation specialist nurses or social workers who took primary responsibility for leading the FDCs in their ICU. This is a modification of current practice and is being evaluated as part of the COMFORT study [4]. Their training was supplemented by simulation training with professional actors through a programme developed and delivered by the NSW Organ and Tissue Donation Service (OTDS) and the Faculty of Health at the University of Technology Sydney [5].

What did we do?

The programme was developed by experts in OTD, intensive care medicine and contemporary simulation techniques. After a two-month planning period, the course was piloted with four members of the development team as participants. Initially the training was in four stages: a telephone conversation with the referring ICU doctor (10 minutes), a planning meeting with the ICU doctor and bedside nurse (15–20 minutes), the FDC with professional actors playing family members (45 minutes) and a three-stage debriefing process (45 minutes, see later). The telephone call was subsequently replaced by a planning sheet in order to save time (see Box 24.1 for an example).

Box 24.1 Planning Meeting Information

This information is provided for the planning meeting with the designated requester, ICU specialist and bedside nurse.
Overview
Simon P is a 24-year-old male
  Assaulted at local pub
  Fell and hit head on concrete, GCS 3 at the scene
  Intubated at scene by ambulance team
  CT scan at the hospital showed a large subdural haemorrhage and base of skull fracture

Decompressive craniectomy and insertion of intracranial pressure (ICP) monitor was performed
  High ICP persisted, repeat CT brain revealed extensive areas of infarction
  Patient was very unstable initially, but was now stable on moderate treatment support

Length of Stay in ICU
5 days

Cause of Death/Impending Death
Intracerebral haemorrhage with extensive infarction

Brain Death Testing Status
Not brain dead

Donation Pathway
Donation after circulatory determination of death

Organ Donor Register
Organs only (not tissues)

Police/Coroners and Forensic Pathologist Involvement
Authorization from coroner and forensic pathologist pending discussion with family

Medical Status
Noradrenaline 4 mg in 100 ml 5% dextrose at 9 ml/hr, vasopressin 2.4 units/hr, desmopressin 0.5 mcg x 2 doses, routine antibiotics, 0.9% saline intravenous infusion

Past Medical History
Nil

Social History
Studying dentistry at university
  Casual work at a dental practice
  Good social network of friends
  Drinks socially, non-smoker, no drugs

Cultural/Religious Background
Christian – non-practising

Family Situation/Dynamics
Lives with twin brother (James) in a Sydney apartment
  James works in finance with Westpac investment branch
  Was with James and other friends at time of the incident
  Parents (Paul and Sarah) live on the NSW north coast
  Family very close and supportive, shocked and traumatized

Family Present in Hospital
Paul, Sarah, James

Conversation Flow
Family has not raised issue of organ donation

Real, anonymized cases were used. In all scenarios, the family had been told that their loved one had received a neurological determination of death (was 'brain dead') or could not survive. The actors were experienced in medical role-play simulation and debriefing, and one of the more experienced actors was a mentor to the others. They were given a synopsis of the scenario and a character brief that included their background, personality, state of mind and the level of emotional intensity, dependent on how the scenario was handled by the participant. They were also provided with a guide to the intended debriefing process. The actors prepared with prior rehearsal and by creating backstories to develop their characters. On the day, they were accommodated in a separate area so that they had no prior contact with the participants and could get into character.

The training was conducted in the university simulation centre with full audio-visual (AV) capabilities, including the ability to annotate scenario recordings. Programme participants and actors signed a consent form for AV recording and to maintain confidentiality. Participants were pre-briefed about the structure of the day and the FDC. They were encouraged to offer support, answer questions and take their time, only raising OTD when they thought the family was ready. They were advised to conduct an engaged conversation on the subject rather than merely impart information, with the overall aim of the family making an informed, proactive decision.

Participants were grouped in pairs, with each observing the other's (different) scenario from the viewing room and then participating in the other's debriefing session.

The planning meeting was held first, with the facilitator playing the ICU doctor. This was followed by an informal debriefing to reflect on the conduct and content of the meeting and cover any information that the participant had missed.

There was a short break while the bedside nurse (played by a senior OTDS staff member) settled the family into the meeting area. The ICU doctor (played

by the facilitator) then led the participant into the room and introduced them to the family in the manner they had requested in the planning meeting. The facilitator then left the room to view and annotate the scenario. When the participant concluded the FDC, or it came to a natural end, the facilitator entered the room unobtrusively and took a seat in the group. They then facilitated a three-stage debriefing process, using the advocacy-with-inquiry model to initiate discussion and reflect on practice [6]. Feedback was first sought from the family in character, to garner initial reactions and emotions. At the discretion of the facilitator, the family and bedside nurse were directed to come out of character to offer further feedback. The actors were then excused and the participant, facilitator and OTDS staff member proceeded to a final debriefing session, in which video-reflexive feedback was used to trigger insight and reflection on practice. A digital file of the participant's video recording was provided for ongoing personal reflection.

After the session, participants completed anonymous evaluation forms specifically created for the programme in which the training was rated using Likert scales, and additional feedback sought via free-text responses.

Various 'escape routes' were integrated to make the training run smoothly. For example, if a participant felt the family needed a break, they could arrange this and leave the room. The actors could then be briefed that a certain time had elapsed so that the conversation could be resumed. If the conversation had not been concluded within an hour, the facilitator entered the room to bring it to a close. This was a very rare occurrence during the training.

What was the impact?

From October 2012 to June 2015, 25 sessions were conducted with 80 participants. DRs were encouraged to repeat the training every 12–18 months: nine participants completed the course twice and one three times.

Evaluation was overwhelmingly positive, with the vast majority of participants expressing that the training was a valuable addition to the PEP. The most frequently cited positive aspects of the training were realistic scenarios using professional actors, feedback on performance and debriefing with peers. Some participants reported that they did not like being observed by others or watching their video recording, but understood the necessity. Participants found video-reflexive feedback especially useful for identifying areas for improvement in body language, phraseology, pace of conversation and missed opportunities to build rapport and display empathy

The majority of participants stated that the training would have a positive effect on their practice, the most commonly cited reasons being consolidation of knowledge, experiential learning using realistic scenarios and building confidence through practice.

Following the introduction of the PEP and simulation training, the family consent rate has risen from 50% to 61% in NSW [7, 8]. Whether the simulation training contributed to this increase is unclear. The COMFORT study is evaluating the effectiveness of this 'best practice' intervention in terms of the effect on family consent rates and whether decisions are enduring [4].

What lessons were learnt?

Following the pilot course, the training was modified to address some limitations, enhance realism and maximize the time available for the FDC and debriefing.

After some initial problems, the actors were given further education about the difficult concept of brain death, because they were supposed to understand this prior to the FDC. The actors' guides were enhanced to provide better information about the potential donor and the characters of the family members. The actors were encouraged to 'reset' after each scenario because of an observed tendency for their behaviour to change over repeated scenarios.

The initial telephone call was removed from the training, because early feedback suggested that it was unnecessary and that more benefit could be derived from increased time for the FDC and debriefing.

The three-stage debriefing process was popular with participants. The comments made by the family while still in character were thought especially useful. There is controversy over whether actors should give feedback in character due to concerns that adverse interactions might be carried forward into the debriefing session [9]. This did not seem to be a problem during our training, which we believe was due to pre-briefing of the actors to give feedback in a sensitive manner and clearly announcing when the actors should come out of character to give further feedback.

We believe that the use of professional actors was a major factor in the success of our programme, with all participants reporting full and immediate immersion in their scenario. We believe that this level of fidelity should be the gold standard for difficult conversations such as the FDC.

There is a growing body of evidence that specialized training in conducting the FDC results in a higher family consent rate and more enduring decisions [10, 11]. Our participants reported increased knowledge and confidence in leading FDCs and all found the training valuable. Whether our training programme contributed to the increased family consent rate seen in NSW over the same period remains unclear. Further insights about the impact of training on subsequent performance during FDC conversations may be gained from follow-up interviews with the clinician participants and from the results of the COMFORT study [4].

References

1 A World's Best Practice Approach to Organ and Tissue Donation for Transplantation. Australian Government, 2008.

2 DonateLife. Clinical Governance Framework, 2013. Available: http://www.donatelife.gov.au/sites/default/files/DonateLife%20Clinical%20Governance%20Framework_0.pdf.

3 Donate Life. Professional Education Package. Available: http://www.donatelife.gov.au/the-authority/education/professional-education-package.

4 Communication with Families regarding Organ and Tissue Donation after Death in Intensive Care Study. Available: https://www.anzctr.org.au/Trial/Registration/TrialReview.aspx?id=364549.

5 UTS Newsroom. Requesting the Gift of Life. April 2014. Available: http://newsroom.uts.edu.au/news/2014/04/requesting-the-gift-of-life?utm_source=life_gk6&utm_medium=gk&utm_ca.

6 Rudolph JW, Simon R, Rivard P, Dufresne RL, Raemer DB. Debriefing with good judgment: combining rigorous feedback with genuine inquiry. *Anesthesiol Clin.* 2007;**25**(2):361–76. PubMed PMID: 17574196.

7 Australian Government Organ and Tissue Authority. Performance report 2010. Available: http://www.donatelife.gov.au/sites/default/files/files/2010_Performance_Report.pdf.

8 Australian Government Organ and Tissue Authority. Performance report 2014. Available: http://www.donatelife.gov.

au/sites/default/files/OTA%202014%20Performance%20Report%20Jan%202015%20FINAL.pdf

9 Nestel, D, Bearman, M, Fleishman, C. (2014) Simulated patients as teachers: the role of feedback. In: Nestel D, Bearman M (Eds). *Simulated Patient Methodology: Theory, Evdence and Practice*, John Wiley & Sons.

10 Vincent A, Logan L. Consent for organ donation. *Br J Anaesth*. 2012;**108**(Suppl 1):i80–i87. PubMed PMID: 22194436.

11 Simpkin AL, Robertson LC, Barber VS, Young JD. Modifiable factors influencing relatives' decision to offer organ donation: systematic review. *BMJ*. 2009;**338**:b991. PubMed PMID: 19383730.

CHAPTER 25

Commencing a simulation-based curriculum in a medical school in China: Independence and integration

Fei Han

Overview

Simulation-based education(SBE) is a complete system, in which the curriculum is an important part – more important than equipment purchasing and facility construction. Our simulation-based medical curriculum philosophy is based on a gradual, repeated and spiral educational format. The curriculum is divided into early contact with clinical course content, clinical experimental courses and intensive training days in three stages before an internship. Compared with other basic and clinical medical school curricula, students from the simulated clinical competence–based curriculum can graduate from the first day to school, then extended to residency training and specialist physician whole-life career training.

A state-of-the-art healthcare simulation facility is ready, and the next step is to see who uses it and how to use it. The curriculum is one of the driving forces of the facility and the investment in equipment provides opportunity for the centre to be an important part of the educational system.

What was the need?

Simulation-based medical training is directly related to the future physician's clinical skill. In the new era, the medical service faces more complicated situations than ever before. The physician needs diverse skills – they are a sociologist with professional medical knowledge and perform professional services. A qualified physician (including all medical staff) plays three roles: clinician, patient educator and resource manager.

As a clinician, doctors need to focus on the technical aspects of medicine, including recognition of patients' risk factors, accurate diagnosis, specific diagnosis, timely diagnosis, appropriate treatment, monitoring and rehabilitation. As a patient educator, the focus needs to be more on the pedagogical aspects of medicine, including having patients understand their illness, having patients understand their treatment, education of the family and education of the wider community. And as a resource manager, doctors need to focus on some of the managerial and financial aspects of medicine, including appropriate utilization of resources. Following our understanding of the contemporary role of the doctor, we developed a simulation-based training system as a platform that integrated medical knowledge with clinical skills, and featured attitudes and behaviours as

Healthcare Simulation Education: Evidence, Theory and Practice, First Edition.
Edited by Debra Nestel, Michelle Kelly, Brian Jolly and Marcus Watson.
© 2018 John Wiley & Sons Ltd. Published 2018 by John Wiley & Sons Ltd.

integral to clinical practice. The goal of the programme goes beyond traditional clinical skill training to improve the future physician's comprehensive competence and build ability and talent in the medical profession.

What did we do?

A six-year medical education programme is popular in Asia. Medical students come from high school, not college. As a pioneer of international medical education in China, Tianjin Medical University developed an independent six-year 500-hour systemic simulation-based training curriculum, and has become a leader in contemporary medical education since 2010. The Integrated simulation-based clinical training curriculum is systemic and continual from the start of medical school through to graduation. The simulation-based curriculum in Tianjin Medical University had Dr Joseph Gonnella, Jefferson Medical College, Philadelphia, USA as an advisor and has been used as a foundation for our medical school curriculum from 2010. Detailed information may be found at http://simhosp.tmu.edu.cn. The skill training timetable aligns with theory in the traditional curriculum. Our simulation-based programme progresses step by step, repeatedly in a spiral educational system. Each step of the training programme is repeated at least three times, and each instance of training has a different focus and purpose, with increasing complexity using a variety of mannequins and task trainers.

In 2010, Tianjin Medical University built a 20,000 square foot simulation hospital (SimHospital) that included recreations of all the hospital facilities relevant to the new curriculum. The facility include a surgical theatre, intensive care unit (ICU), outpatient rooms, inpatient rooms, obstetric delivery rooms, gynaecology training room, paediatric training room, registration window and nurse stations. All of the training rooms can be set up as objective structured clinical examination (OSCE) stations with wi-fi camera and one-way transforming windows. Additionally, there is an outdoor emergency training field. The facility is a replica of the hospital, using sophisticated mannequins and simulated patients instead of real patients. Essential basic clinical skill training needs are addressed, including teamwork training, medical communication, case-writing skills and medical attitude training.

Simulation-based training was started at same time as the SimHospital was completed. Five hundred hours of simulation-based clinical skills training were embedded in the curriculum using a staged approach:

- *Basic medical lecture stage (first three years, 138 hours)*: This early exposure to medical training focuses on basic clinical concepts, medical ethics, the art of medical writing and communication, basic team work, physical examination, trauma treatment, patient transfer, basic surgical technique, cardiopulmonary resuscitation (CPR) and hospital visiting. The purpose of this stage of training is to give medical students one whole medical service image, even though some training topics will be taught formally in future classes. However, we still introduce these topics early in the medical course because students have to know that they are a doctor already, and understand that what they learn will make a difference to or save people's lives. Understanding professional attitudes is important for students when they enter medical school.

- *Clinical lecture stage (next two years, 122 hours)*: Training includes clinical skills and team work with real clinical cases. Immediately after the clinical lecture, students practise the same content with the simulator in the simulation facility. Each class of 30 students is divided into groups of 3–6 practising the content at the same time in the same or different rooms. Now when students study the basic medical sciences, a new period of laboratory experiments follows the lectures. We wanted students to have a similar learning experience after lectures in the clinical courses rather than, or in addition to, going straight into the hospital. In keeping with the same learning format as the basic science courses, we named the new simulation facility-based training course the 'clinical experiment course'. Students come to the simulation facility after clinical lectures and the training content tightly matches what they have just been taught.

- *Pre-internship stage (the end of the fifth year)*: Medical students have a concentrated 8 weeks, 200 hours of self-clinical skill training in the simulation facility before their internship starts, including real clinical scenarios incorporating medical teamwork, behaviour and clinical skills. they review all the technical and non-technical skills that they have learnt in the previous five years, from medical writing, medical communication and professional skills, through to critical care team work and advanced emergency training. Training is guided and graded by the teaching faculty and includes general knowledge via lectures, bedside teaching and practice grading. All students' practice is recorded by video, and students have a group debriefing using the recorded video footage without the supervisor's guidance. At the same time, supervisors also may be grading students' performance using the same video-recorded material. In total, a student may practise 12 disease cases within a clinical scenario incorporating simulated patients to learn all the related skills. After the complete scenario-based examination, successful students will achieve approval to transition from medical student to doctor.

• *Internship stage (the sixth year)*: Students will learn and practise with real patients. SimHospital provides the final department skill examination only.

A simulation-based education (SBE) platform is a template, involving various traditional teaching topics and subjects together, especially medical students' attitude training. In a traditional curriculum, attitude training may be a separate course or be learnt from a senior physician, while a simulation-based curriculum provides an individual experience. Developing professional attitudes is also integrated into each clinical skill training class. In our university, the clinical skill training curriculum had been expanded to a 'clinical abilitology' course. Medical ethics, medical law, medical communication, drug development and medical history have been incorporated into the simulation-based curriculum to improve a medical student's comprehensive medical competence.

A simulation-based curriculum is normally supported by a simulation facility, and it does not matter whether the facility is independent or in situ. Students are the chief actors. Video camera, wi-fi connection and Google Glass provide more opportunities and methods to enable students to practise alone with remote guidance from supervisors. Students may play the role of an independent physician or a member of a medical team in any of the training stages, and also role play as physician and nurse and so on. Group discussion and debriefing will be held after every practice case under faculty guidance. A unique benefit of simulation-based training is the integration of theory with practice. Students deal with simulated patients and simulate real clinical cases, practise in the SimHospital, a replica of a real clinical environment,

and do scenarios, role play and self-debriefing. Using these strategies, students find the problem, discuss and solve the problem and find new problems, improving their self-learning competence step by step.

The difficulty of an SBE curriculum is how to integrate it into the traditional Chinese medical curriculum. Tianjin Medical University developed a 500-hour simulation-based curriculum and 200–300 hours of clinical training integrated with the traditional curriculum, built the template to incorporate some subjects into the new curriculum, and aligned simulation-based lab practice with traditional lectures. Baby delivery is one sample course:

• Baby delivery I: Classroom lecture
• Baby delivery II: learn baby delivery movement with simple simulator in SimHospital
• Baby delivery III: learn whole baby delivery procedure with high-level simulator
• Baby delivery IV: learn postpartum complications in ICU, SimHospital

A new curriculum needs to increase the teaching hours, which increases the burden on students and faculty. We tried to integrate the new curriculum into the classic courses, which improved the traditional teaching effect without increasing the teaching hours.

What was the impact?

The new simulation-based medical curriculum was implemented in Tianjin Medical University over four years. Simulation-based medical training is new in all medical schools in China, and even worldwide. Different countries and schools will face different situations and challenges, and we believe that no standardized curriculum can meet everyone's needs. Self-evaluation and improvement systems for local needs are necessary for all curricula. Surveys of students and faculty, and knowledge examination and internship performance data analysis, are important to determine whether the new curriculum is successful and to identify areas for improvement.

What lessons were learnt?

An ideal simulation-based medical curriculum is a comprehensive training platform (Figure 25.1) founded

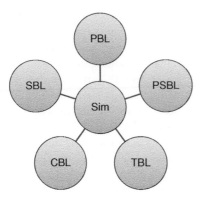

Figure 25.1 Simulation-based training may involve all of the teaching methods. CBL = case-based learning, PBL = problem-based learning, PSBL = problem solving–based learning, SBL = scenario-based learning, TBL = team-based learning.

on case-based learning (CBL), in the form of team-based learning (TBL), in the space of scenario-based learning (SBL), directed by problem-based learning (PBL), with the final goal of problem solving–based learning (PSBL). With collaborative curriculum development based on contemporary educational techniques, physicians and simulation experts need to cooperate closely, and at the same time introduce modern technology into teaching and learning approaches at different stages. Longstanding, traditional curricula can be modified to include contemporary training to produce doctors who can meet the challenges required of them in modern healthcare settings.

Acknowledgement

I am especially grateful to Dr Joseph Gonnella, Jefferson Medical College, Philadelphia, USA. All of my knowledge of medical education was obtained from him when I worked in Jefferson. I brought his ideas to this chapter and implanted them in my work in China.

CHAPTER 26

Transport of the critically ill patient: Developing safe practices

Rafidah Atan, Kristian Krogh, Nor'azim Mohd Yunos, Suneet Sood, Naganathan & Debra Nestel

---

KEY MESSAGES

- Transporting the critically ill patient is an important skill for doctors.

- Simulation can be used to develop safe practices in transporting critically ill patients.

- Component skills and knowledge are essential to maximize the integrated simulation activity.

- Simulation is an excellent tool for medical students and interns in transporting critically ill patients, as it combines experiential learning with a high degree of support.

Overview

In this chapter we describe a programme using immersive simulation to support the development of safe practices in transport of the critically ill patient. The programme, which was successful in obtaining a curriculum development grant from Monash University, addresses intrahospital transport and is offered to final-year medical students in Malaysia. The consolidation of the programme involved inputs from clinicians and educationalists from both local and international arenas.

What was the need?

The objective of medical training is to produce safe and competent doctors whose tasks are determined by local policies. Transporting critically ill patients exposes patients to adverse events even when conducted by experts [1]. In our context, this skill has previously been developed through first-hand experience. This trial-and-error approach is no longer acceptable, especially with the wide availability of simulation tools. In developing countries new doctors may be required to transport critically ill patients independently, which further increases the threat to patient safety. Therefore, we developed a simulation-based education (SBE) programme to support the development of safe practices in the transport of critically ill patients for final-year medical students.

High fidelity immersive simulation is an ideal tool for this purpose, as it provides an experiential learning opportunity in a *patient*-safe environment [2]. Learning by 'doing' engages learners better, compared to classroom activities or unguided passive observations in the clinical environment [3].

Preparation and equipment use during the transport of patients may not always meet safety standards due to constraints, but also due to a lack of awareness. Simulation allows medical students to be introduced to standards of care and monitoring that should be met during transport, so that they can initiate this important change for the future. The reflective process of experiential learning helps participants to develop awareness when next observing or participating in the transport of ill patients.

As patient transportation is difficult and complex, an extensive set of prior learning and basic skills are required of participants for the simulation session to have maximum benefit.

What did we do?

The programme

Final-year medical students in the emergency medicine rotation in Monash University Malaysia are offered the programme. Although the medical curriculum contains a compulsory unit on patient safety, this module was developed as an extension to reflect local needs.

The main objective of the programme is for students to demonstrate safe transport of a critically ill patient, including:

- Adequate preparation prior to transport
- Adequate monitoring of the patient during transport
- Safe handover of care to the receiving team

Adequate preparation includes knowing the patient's medical background, ensuring stability for transfer and packing adequate equipment and drugs for the journey. Adequate monitoring includes full monitoring equipment and constant vigilance, despite distractions that will occur during the transport, followed by correct management of unstable parameters. Safe handover includes correct identification of essential information that needs to be communicated, including events that occurred during the transport.

At the start of the rotation, students are instructed to undertake self-directed learning activities including readings, careful observation of transport of patients in the clinical environment and discussions with clinical staff to gain insight. Readings are adapted from a professional document [4]. This is a specific instruction given to students at the start of the rotation to prepare them for the simulation session. We find that if this instruction is not given, students tend to skip these important steps.

Prior to participation in the programme, students attend three full days of the original Monash patient safety unit. This includes interactive tutorials, workshops and immersive simulation scenarios. Relevant elements of patient safety, human error, team work and communication are emphasized. The immersive simulation scenarios, including an advanced cardiac life support training session, introduce students to crisis management principles and the rules of engagement in simulation activities. Students are taught a standard approach in managing deteriorating patients following the acronym ABCDE, which is similar to the Advanced Trauma Life Support (ATLS) algorithm [5]. Students are also taught a standard format for making phone referrals and giving verbal handovers, which

they further practise during the scenarios. These prior experiences contribute to a safe learning environment for the students and a high level of engagement.

Incidentally, the patient safety unit classes are quite extensive. These are more than briefings: students undergo three full days (8 a.m. to 6 p.m.) of patient safety sessions, which drive home these learning points on human error, team work and communication, and crisis management. We believe that the classes added significantly to the fact that our students were somewhat ready for the difficult skill of transporting an ill patient. The patient safety and crisis management sessions helped the students attain a certain level of maturity in handling ill patients. If it had not been for these prior learning experiences, the cognitive load might have been too great for them.

In a one-hour interactive tutorial, a transport-oriented variation of the acronym DRSABCDE is introduced (Figure 26.1). The acronym is designed as a simple mental checklist that will help students fulfil the objectives of a safe transport. Students then apply the acronym while working through three problem-based scenarios during the tutorial: a patient who appears stable but is at risk of sudden deterioration; a second patient who is clearly critically ill – intubated, with a vasopressor infusion and a chest tube; and a third patient who is too unstable for transfer.

During the transport simulation session, a group of approximately five students first prepare a transport bag and all of its contents. The students then demonstrate transport of a high-fidelity mannequin, in the context of a clinical scenario, within the compounds of the medical school to mimic intrahospital transport (Figure 26.2). During the transport, patient parameters deteriorate, challenging the students first to detect the deterioration and then to institute basic measures as a response. On arrival at the destination, the patient deteriorates further, so that students are aware of this particular danger period, when an untrained transporting team lowers their guard before continuity of care is ensured or handed over. At the end of the transfer students have to perform a verbal handover to the receiving doctor.

The performance of the task includes debriefing components, both in-simulation (pause and discuss) [6] and post-simulation. The patient transported corresponds to one of the tutorial scenarios so that students are cognizant of potential issues. Sessions take approximately 90 minutes.

D	*Is the patient stable for transfer?* Check vital signs stat. Get to know the patient.
R	*Check response*
S	*Do I need help?*
A	*Assess airway* Bring equipment/drugs to support airway.
B	*Assess breathing* Bring equipment/drugs to support breathing.
C	*Assess circulation* Bring equipment/drugs to support circulation.
D	*Assess disability* Bring equipment/drugs to support disability.
E	*Assess environment* Manage environment to facilitate safe transfer.

Figure 26.1 Transport-oriented variation of the acronym DRSABCDE.

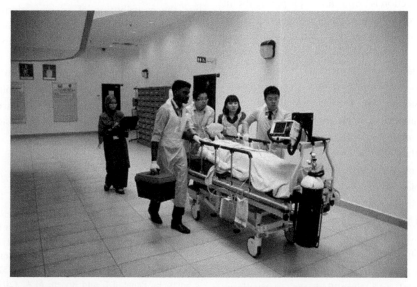

Figure 26.2 Students transporting a mannequin around the clinical school accompanied by a facilitator.

Students are accompanied by an instructor. Unsafe practices invite a 'pause' followed by a short debriefing/instruction in the correct practice in order to minimize erroneous take-home points [7, 8]. As medical students have few real clinical experiences, there is a higher risk of negative learning when only using post-simulation debriefing, as errors in practice are not corrected immediately, including errors that do not appear to lead to an adverse event. We also anticipate multiple errors by the students, making it difficult to debrief them all during post-simulation debriefing. In-simulation debriefing also provides support to students when they are facing uncertainty on how to progress.

Students are again debriefed at the conclusion of the session, during which a summary of safe practices for transporting critically ill patients is again outlined. The contents of the transport bag that the students have prepared are compared to a checklist and feedback given regarding their adequacy.

What was the impact?

The various components of the programme were designed to help students continue to reflect following the learning encounter, generate interest in the subject matter and heighten their insight when next observing or participating in the transport of ill patients in the clinical environment. A pre and post questionnaire on knowledge and attitude is also part of the programme as an added effort to stimulate interest and reflection. Since the programme is only offered once for each student, this continued reflection is important in preparing them for their future role. The multiple learning activities associated with this module are also in keeping with the faculty's move to implement blended learning in the curriculum and may encourage deep learning.

Embedding this programme in our curriculum was aided by its inclusion as part of the emergency medicine rotation. Some acute medicine tutorial topics such as cardiac arrest algorithm, oxygen therapy and fluid management further help to prepare the students. The compulsory patient safety unit ensured that extensive prior learning topics are covered.

Following the initial implementation, we have further consolidated the programme. This process mainly involved simplification of the learning points that students must attain by the end of the transport session. For example, we have shortened the case scenarios during the tutorial and simplified the instructions accompanying the DRSABCDE acronym. We have also scheduled specific times during which the acronym is reiterated: during the tutorial while discussing case scenarios, at the start of the transport simulation session and at the final debriefing session. Some of these insights were obtained following consultation with international colleagues who teach transport of critically ill patients via formal national training programmes in their country.

What lessons were learnt?

There were three key lessons. First, when the module was piloted, we did not include a tutorial component. Students were instructed to acquire theoretical knowledge only through self-directed learning activities prior to the simulation session. However, students found the simulation session overwhelming, with too many insights to grasp at once. It seemed obvious that the cognitive load was too great [9]. An interactive tutorial session was subsequently introduced, prior to the simulation session, to allow a detailed discussion of the topic including a specific discussion of the case; that is, the patient who was to be transported during the simulation session. We found that this addition significantly increased the quality of the experience. This could be further enhanced by a live or video demonstration prior to the simulation session. What was important was the opportunity to consolidate knowledge prior to the simulation. A second lesson was the contribution of an educational development grant from the university, which was a trigger to focus our attention on addressing an educational need in our curriculum. The grant also provided us with an avenue to promote this topic of study at the faculty level. A third lesson was the value of consulting colleagues outside of our immediate workplace to share international perspectives on practice and to gain insight into further consolidation of the programme.

References

1 Beckmann, U., Gillies, D.M., Berenholtz, S.M., Wu, A.W., Pronovost, P. (2004) Incidents relating to the intra-hospital transfer of critically ill patients. An analysis of the reports submitted to the Australian Incident Monitoring Study in Intensive Care. *Intensive Care Med*, **30**(8):1579–85.

2 Salas, E., Paige, J.T. and Rosen, M.A. (2013) Creating new realities in healthcare: the status of simulation-based training as a patient safety improvement strategy. *BMJ Qual Saf*, **22** (6), 449–52.

3 Okuda, Y., Bryson, E.O., DeMaria, S. Jr., *et al.* (2009) The utility of simulation in medical education: what is the evidence? *Mt Sinai J Med*, **76** (4), 330–43.

4 Australian and New Zealand College of Anaesthetists. Guidelines for transport of critically ill patients, November 2013 [cited 16 September 2016]. Available at: http://www.anzca .edu.au/documents/ps52-2015-guidelines-for-transport-of-critically-i.pdf

5 American College of Surgeons. Advanced trauma life support [cited 9 September 2015]. Available at: https://www.facs.org/quality%20programs/trauma/atls

6 Hogan, J., Flanagan, B. and Marshall, S. (2008) What facilitation skills and behaviours optimise students' learning when using a simulator in the 'pause and discuss' mode? *Focus Health Prof Educ*, **10** (2), 36–7.

7 Curtis, M.T., DiazGranados, D. and Feldman, M. (2012) Judicious use of simulation technology. *Contin Med Educ*, **32** (4), 255–60.

8 Krogh, K.B., Høyer, C.B., Ostergaard, D. and Eika, B. (2014) Time matters: realism in resuscitation training. *Resuscitation*, **85** (8), 1093–8.

9 van Merrienboer, J. and Sweller, J. (2010) Cognitive load theory in health professional education: design principles and strategies. *Med Educ*, **44** (1), 85–93.

CHAPTER 27

From routine to leadership: Extending the role of simulation technicians in Southeast Asia

Bee Leng Sabrina Koh & Chaoyan Dong

KEY MESSAGES

- The turnover of experienced simulation technicians in Southeast Asia is high.
- High turnover has a significant impact on the continuity of simulation centre operations.
- The current career path of a simulation technician stops at being a technician.
- Simulation technicians' roles can be extended to include teaching responsibilities and to lead training of the next generation of technicians.

Overview

In Asia, experienced simulation technicians are rare, and the mechanism for simulation centres to train technicians is not well established. Very often simulation technicians are recruited with diplomas in engineering or information technology (IT) and receive on-the-job training in simulation applications. The job title is often classified as *training laboratory assistant* or *technical support* staff, without a clear career path that can potentially evolve into a recognized specialist role appropriate to the field. Also, well-developed simulation training programmes are required to prepare technicians for the job. The skills include audio-visual technology, hardware and software application, basic understanding of health professional education and management of the learning environment. These skills can be transferred and applied to other industries, for example, multimedia

broadcasting, healthcare equipment manufacturing and healthcare education systems. Based on our experience, many technicians who were trained in simulation have left to pursue a career in other industries after a brief stint in healthcare simulation. Therefore, it is important for institutions to develop retention strategies to maximize their efforts and keep operations on track. This case study describes our experience in developing a specific retention strategy to facilitate technicians' transition towards assuming extended roles.

What was the need?

In most simulation centres, technicians have quite different responsibilities compared to simulation educators. Technicians have a unique set of competencies and are required to demonstrate these skills. The ideal technician should also be willing to take long-term ownership of and responsibility for the job, but due to the limited prospects for career progression, many soon leave for more attractive careers in other industries.

The departure of these technicians can significantly affect simulation centre operations and lower other staff's morale. A new recruit cannot fully replace the trained technician initially, and financial and time investments are required to train the newly hired technician to acquire the competencies needed to operate independently. To train newly hired technicians, the simulation educators may need to reschedule classes, step in to cover the technician's role and, in the worst

Healthcare Simulation Education: Evidence, Theory and Practice, First Edition.
Edited by Debra Nestel, Michelle Kelly, Brian Jolly and Marcus Watson.
© 2018 John Wiley & Sons Ltd. Published 2018 by John Wiley & Sons Ltd.

case, postpone courses. A technician's departure can be multifaceted and have impacts on the centre, simulation educators, learners and the institution.

Most technicians who resigned cited the lack of role development along with stagnation in job scope. It has become a common understanding that prompt corrective actions avert more critical situations. So further development of the technician role became the focus in the hope of improved job satisfaction and retention.

In response to the known disruptions and reasons already cited, we explored the possibility of expanding the career path for simulation technicians, to learn to become a technician educator. This career path offered simulation technicians additional opportunities beyond their normal roles, such as a level of sub-specialist expertise, a leadership role, serving as a mentor for novice technicians, and involvement in specific research projects. If this initiative proved to be successful, simulation centres would retain experienced technicians through extending their roles to being educators, mentors and researchers to develop novice technicians.

What did we do?

The Simulation Technician/Specialist Development Programme (STSDP) commenced in 2009 as an in-house induction course in a Singapore hospital and was developed to train newly hired technicians. The four modules (Table 27.1) were developed for participants with little or no healthcare background to achieve job competency as a simulation technician.

The course objectives mirror the scope of the job. The general learning outcomes included:

- Design and programme a clinical scenario for use in simulation programmes.
- Facilitate learning in simulation through efficient technical support and management.

- Manage a simulation facility: data storage and equipment care.

The course modules consist of structured didactic, self-directed learning packages, technical skills stations, role play, return demonstration and executing a learner's designed simulated activity. The course instructors were nurse educators experienced in simulation.

The STSDP modules were well received, so the programme was extended to overseas participants, including technicians and educators from Indonesia, the Philippines, Thailand, India and Malaysia. We soon realized that our faculty team could not meet the increasing demand for the programme, as they had to juggle their clinical duties and teaching. We decided to recruit technicians who graduated from the programme to teach, and helped them to develop towards a teaching role. One benefit for technicians serving as faculty is that they can share first-hand experiences with participants during teaching. The final impact is better because it potentially frees nurse educators from a heavy teaching load so they still can fulfil their clinical duties. In our first trial, the programme was entrusted to two experienced senior technicians who had graduated from the programme, one from Singapore and one from Malaysia.

To prepare the two candidates to take on the faculty role, they were invited to observe and co-facilitate the course with senior nurse educators. These nurse educators were experienced in teaching the course and provided mentorship for the two candidates, including sharing insights into faculty roles and responsibilities, requirements, commitment, time management and intellectual property management. The technicians were also given the task of managing the website through which course materials such as powerpoint slides, reading materials, learning packages and assignments are circulated with a password (Figure 27.1). The online materials are given to registered participants as

Table 27.1 STSDP modules.

Module	Title	Lecture/ tutorial	Workshop/ practice	Total hours
1	Simulation Technician/Specialist: Scope of Work	6	–	6
2	Introduction to Healthcare Simulation and Modalities	8	10	18
3	Simulation Equipment and Accessories	10	10	20
4	Scenario Programming	12	8	20
Total hours		**36**	**28**	**64**

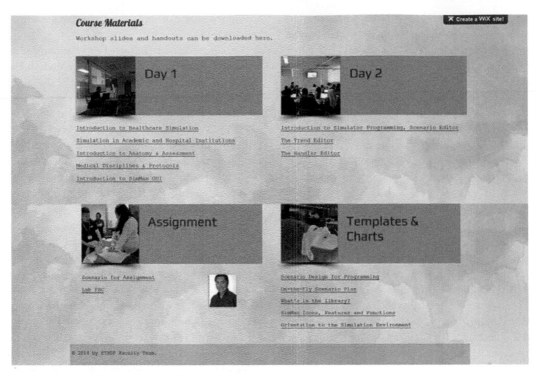

Figure 27.1 Screenshot of the Simulation Technician Course site.

preparation for the work that needs to be done in class. Pre-download of assignments and files that complement the assignment is essential to avoid disappointment due to network issues.

A learning package on medical terminology and healthcare basics was provided for participants without a background in the healthcare industry. The aim was to facilitate their understanding of the course materials and the particular dialogue and terms used in this field and required for their role.

Six months later the two candidates were fully in charge of the programme, including course planning, content modification, lecture delivery and evaluation.

What was the impact?

To explore the impact of this initiative on the two technician faculty members, they were invited to share their thoughts and experiences with us. An interview was conducted face to face with the Singapore technician and via email questionnaire with the one in Malaysia, due to geographical limitations. Refer to Appendix 27.1 for the questionnaire items. Responses from the two technician educators are summarized in the following sections.

Confidence in teaching

The observation and co-facilitation of teaching with experienced nurse educators helped them to understand the expectations of being a faculty member, and helped to structure the preparation phase. The exposure to teaching techniques has greatly increased their confidence for subsequent programme delivery and management. Frequent communication with co-faculty and mentors ensured timely answers to their questions during teaching.

Satisfaction

A particular satisfying moment was when they shared experiences in teaching how to manage a high-technology patient simulator, including the features and troubleshooting common glitches. They found that they were able to provide additional insights, since they could demonstrate the full range of simulator features, which are often underutilized. For example, one comment was: 'The learners were discussing at lunch that they are going to replicate our teaching in their institution! This shows that we are doing it the right way.'

Career and self-improvement

Their engagement in teaching has enriched their experience. Both expressed that they will need constantly to maintain and improve their knowledge and to keep abreast of developments in simulation in order to 'remain in the game'. The exposure has also motivated them to develop new simulation scenarios to meet upcoming needs.

Their new role in teaching has enhanced their career prospects and has inspired others to join the workforce. It is a breakthrough in terms of career stasis.

Teaching has provided an extended role and career progression for simulation technicians beyond a monetary level. The development of technician faculty has the potential for growth towards a *technologist specialism* that encompasses a variety of aspects related to supporting and innovating technology within healthcare simulation.

What lessons were learned?

It is a lengthy process for technicians to become competent in healthcare simulation, and to acquire and apply teaching skills to serve as educators. It definitely requires commitment from all parties. The temptation for technicians to move to a different industry is always present and concerns those running simulation facilities. Our strategy has proven effective through getting the institution involved, recognizing simulation technicians' achievements and providing opportunities for extended roles. Institutional recognition of the role and the contribution of the mentors should also be emphasized, because they play a significant role in ensuring the success of the initiative. Through developing and retaining a pool of excellent technicians, the long-term return on investment will be significant. The technicians were able to play a key role in the inaugural pan-Asia simulation conference in late 2015 (see Figure 27.2).

Following on from our local initiative, and in recognition of the need, the Society for Simulation in Healthcare commenced the Certified Healthcare Simulation Operations Specialist programme in 2014. Its purpose is for technicians to get formal recognition for their specialist skills in simulation operations and also to confirm their commitment to the profession. Hopefully institutions will value such a certificate and recognize its benefits. We aim to advocate this same programme through our regional simulation society to increase institutional awareness and buy-in.

One vendor who has established a good working relationship with the faculty team in Asia has been involved

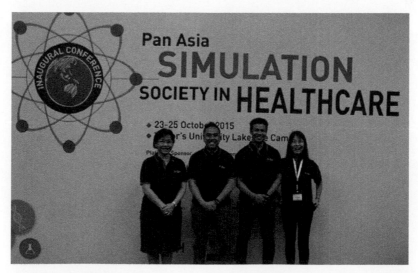

Figure 27.2 The next-generation simulation technicians (centre) and mentors (Sabrina Koh far left and Chaoyan Dong far right). Reproduced with permission.

in publicizing and recruiting participants for similar programmes in Asia. Although the simulators used in the programme have been provided by this vendor, equipment and materials from a variety of vendors need to be incorporated into future programmes. This will help with progressing the course to an advanced level with wider applicability. To prevent perceived conflicts of interest, the faculty team may consider taking on the operational tasks at a regional simulation society level or institutional level on mutually agreed terms.

Conclusion

For successful and uninterrupted operations, it is sensible to develop a group of competent simulation technicians and to provide them with opportunities for continuing professional development to reduce attrition. We hope that our innovative practice in Southeast Asia can inspire others interested in becoming or developing a team of simulation technicians.

Appendix 27.1: Email questionnaire

1 What is your overall impression of having taught in the Sim tech course (STSDP)?
2 What did you envision yourself doing on knowing that you were invited to teach in the STSDP?
3 What were your expectations of being a faculty member (your expectations of the course, preparation, intended outcome)?
4 Please elaborate on the teaching exposure that this course has given you.
5 Were there unexpected events, incidents or occurrences?
6 Were there any satisfying moments? (Or any dissatisfaction?)
7 How do you plan to improve yourself for the next run?
8 Has this exposure affect your career? How?
9 Any other thoughts that you want to express?

CHAPTER 28

Incorporating simulation in a medical city: A case study from King Fahad Medical City

Hani Lababidi

KEY MESSAGES

- Simulation in a medical city is challenging in its scale and specifications.
- Multidisciplinary and longitudinal simulation has a favourable impact on patient safety.
- Simulation can be heavily utilized in system integration and patient experience.

Overview

A medical city is a set of tertiary care hospitals in one geographical location or of the same academic affiliation. Accordingly, simulation in a medical city carries more specifications and challenges when compared to a simulation in a single hospital. This case study will use King Fahad Medical City (KFMC) in Riyadh, Saudi Arabia as a prototype for others who wish to embark on this journey.

Introduction

King Fahad Medical City (KFMC; see Figure 28.1) consists of four hospitals (Main, Children, Women and Rehabilitation), four specialized centres (Cardiac, Cancer, Neurosciences and Endocrine) and a Faculty of Medicine with a total of 1200 beds. The 7600 workers at KFMC are multicultural, with more than 48 nationalities represented. This fact provides unique challenges, but we strongly believe in achieving a uniform approach to patient care through rigorous education and training.

What was the need?

Models of simulation-based education

A simulation program in a medical city can take one of two approaches: it can follow either the segregated or integrated model.

Segregated model

This model is based on establishing different simulation programmes or centres within the medical city and each one works independently. The main driving force for this model would be financial and/or administrative independency of the different simulation centres within the medical city or the university-affiliated hospitals. This model is de facto most of the time and can result in wasting of resources and duplication of work. However, it carries many advantages: it provides a plethora of experience over a wide array of specialisms with healthy competition to achieve excellence, more in-depth research and innovations.

Integrated model

This model is based on establishing one simulation programme for the whole medical city with a central governing body and funding. Within this programme there may be multiple sites that run different simulation activities. The advantage of this model is multifactorial: first, it can be easily aligned with and helps to advance the mission, vision and strategic objectives of the mother institution; second, it reduces duplication of equipment, simulators and supplies.

Healthcare Simulation Education: Evidence, Theory and Practice, First Edition.
Edited by Debra Nestel, Michelle Kelly, Brian Jolly and Marcus Watson.
© 2018 John Wiley & Sons Ltd. Published 2018 by John Wiley & Sons Ltd.

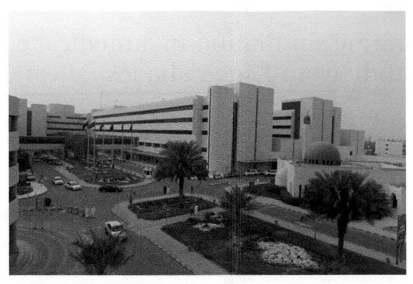

Figure 28.1 Part of King Fahad Medical City complex.

What did we do?

We elected to consolidate all simulation activities at KFMC under one centre: the Center for Research, Education and Simulation Enhanced Training (CRESENT).

All simulation equipment at CRESENT is centrally managed and various simulation sites throughout KFMC can borrow it through an established equipment loan policy and procedure. The simulation centre staff is more easily managed by centralized processes, including hiring, faculty development and promotions. It also allows a uniform methodology for scheduling, conducting and reporting simulation activities that will aid in obtaining accurate data for certification by accreditation bodies.

Organizational governance

There are many structure and governance models for simulation centres that depend heavily on the structure of the mother institution (1). All educational and academic activities at KFMC are governed by the Academic and Training Affairs administration (ATA). The director of CRESENT reports to the executive director of ATA, who in turns reports to the chief executive officer (CEO) of the medical city. There are four departments at CRESENT:

- *Undergraduate Simulation*: This department is charged with all simulation activities related to medical students. While it reports administratively to CRESENT, academically it is governed by the assistant dean for medical education at the Faculty of Medicine.
- *Postgraduate Simulation*: This department is in charge of all simulation-based education (SBE) for clinical and non-clinical healthcare workers at KFMC. Given the huge tasks and challenges of this department, it is assisted by two committees:
  o Allied Health Simulation Committee, which consists of representatives from nursing, pharmacy, respiratory therapy, biomedical engineering, information technology (IT), infection control, administration and hospital security.
  o Residency Programmes Simulation Committee, which comprises representatives from residency and fellowship training programmes.
- *Curriculum Development*: This department is staffed with experts in medical education who aid course directors and instructors in instructional design, curriculum development and curriculum evaluation. An important assignment for this department is to establish simulation curricula for various residencies and fellowship programmes (2).
- *Life Support Training*: This department is responsible for the development and administration of all life support training courses at KFMC.

Types of simulation-based education

According to a Joint Commission report, the most common source of medical errors and breach of patient safety is poor communication among the various healthcare workers throughout the patient journey (3). Most of these errors can be avoided by improving team-work skills, communication, leadership, adherence to protocols and policies, sharing information and moving towards a culture of quality and safety (4). CRESENT simulation programmes offer various kinds of simulation training with a range of complexities. These exercises can be practised in different modalities in order to improve team work and enhance patient safety.

Multidisciplinary simulation

Multidisciplinary simulation training involves a cohort of healthcare providers who commonly work together in the real world. Team training is practised heavily in multidisciplinary simulation, such as team work, situational awareness, communication skills and crisis management (5). It can be structured to include all levels of healthcare workers who are involved in specific patient care processes. The larger the group of specialisms involved, the more challenges there are in terms of conducting the scenario and assessing the cognitive and non-cognitive skills. Examples of such training at CRESENT are postpartum haemorrhage and transcatheter aortic valve implantation (TAVI) modules.

Continuum of care

A great proportion of simulation training is being delivered in a modular fashion. However, in the real world patients are treated by team-based care, as different teams work together throughout the patient's hospitalization journey. Continuum of care or longitudinal simulation is defined as multidisciplinary simulation training to reflect the patient's hospital care pathway. For example, at CRESENT we train cardiology team members in an acute myocardial infarction scenario, from recognition and diagnosis in the emergency department to patient transfer for acute angioplasty in the cardiac catheterization suite and then on to the coronary care unit (CCU).

What was the impact?

Multidepartment simulation

Multidepartment simulation is defined as multidisciplinary training of teams from more than one department in a longitudinal fashion. In an actual hospital environment, there are interactions between departments all the time. For example, a patient admitted to the emergency department (ED) with symptoms of acute stroke would be stabilized after initial assessment by the ED team. Then the care is handed over to the stroke team, with the patient often being transferred to the radiology department for imaging and possible cerebral angiography, and then to the final disposition in the stroke unit. Several key objectives are practised during the journey of such a patient scenario, for example prioritization in the ED, early detection and diagnosis of stroke, effective handover techniques, communication skills, team work and even skills training for endovascular thrombolysis or clot-retrieval techniques.

Non-clinical simulation

Most SBE efforts have been tailored towards clinical staff, namely physicians, nurses, respiratory therapists, paramedics and pharmacists. At CRESENT, there is a holistic approach to SBE to include non-clinical staff as well. This can be achieved through multidisciplinary SBE or stand-alone SBE for various healthcare workers. Examples of non-clinical SBE include uniform practising of key skills pertaining to hospital security such as dealing with violent patients, potential child abduction, bomb threats and disaster management. Further scenarios focus on nutrition and food handling, safe storage, preparation and presentation of food. And finally, housekeeping staff (Figure 28.2) can be made more aware of infection control practices and cleaning techniques for the different surfaces found across hospital departments.

System testing and integration

A valuable use of healthcare simulation is in testing systems prior to commissioning new departments or units in a medical city (6). System integration or operational readiness testing can detect major and minor errors that can affect staff working conditions and hence patient safety in the real world. Two examples can shed light on such processes. Prior to opening a new bronchoscopy

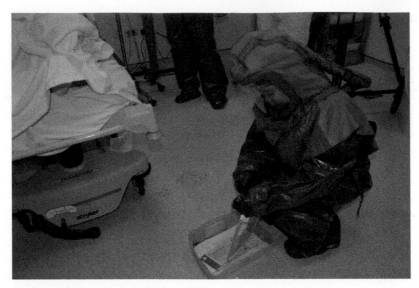

Figure 28.2 Housekeeper trainee, part of multidisciplinary training on Ebola preparedness.

unit, we ran an in-situ simulation using a full body mannequin and a bronchial tree model. The system was tested from scheduling of the procedure to performing the actual bronchoscopy on the model in the presence of all stakeholders. A few minor errors were identified and corrected during the scenario; however, one major issue was that the narcotic cabinet was relatively far away from the endoscopy room and the nurse had to leave the patient unattended for a few minutes in order to get more narcotics. As a result, the narcotic cabinet was moved to a closer location. Another example related to the computed tomography (CT) scan suite, where a mock patient code was simulated on the CT table. The suction outlet was positioned on the wall behind the CT machine and the suction tubing was not long enough to reach the head of the mannequin, so portable suction equipement had to be utilized. The system error was immediately corrected by placing extension suction tubing in the crash cart and making it a regularly checked item.

Patient experience simulation

An innovative programme at CRESENT is the use of simulation to improve the patient experience and thus patient and family satisfaction. It is achieved through enhancing patient and family learning experience and familiarizing them with medical practices and procedures. For example, patients were acquainted with the concept of a 'time-out' in the operating theatre

through an awareness campaign, where an operating room replica was made in the lobby of the main hospital and patients with scheduled surgeries as well as the general public were invited to engage with the set-up. A team from anaesthesia and surgery departments explained the concept with enactments. In another occasion, mock-up magnetic resonance imaging (MRI) with sound effects was used to simulate the patient experience. Recently, one ICU room, out of the 75 adult ICU beds at KFMC, has been converted to an in-situ simulation room with a SimMan 3G® mannequin. A programme is being developed in conjunction with the departments of critical care medicine and health education to familiarize family members of ICU patients with the environment, with special attention paid to infection control precautions. Families of ICU patients will be taken to this room and a health educator will demonstrate to them the various 'hardware' they are likely to see, such as intravenous (IV) lines, tubes, ventilators and syringe pumps. The ICU team utilizes the room for in-situ simulations as well.

What lessons were learnt?

The concept of a simulation hospital

CRESENT is in the process of advancing simulation in the medical city to a new frontier. There are plans to establish a simulation hospital in the near future.

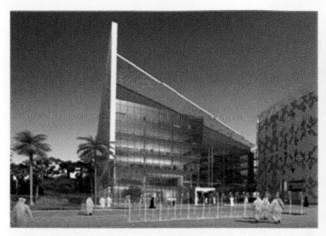 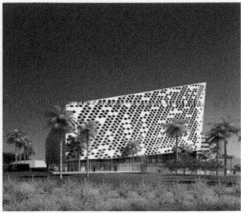

Figure 28.3 Sketches of the future Simulation Hospital at King Fahad Medical City.

CRESENT is moving into a new 22,000 square metre (237,000 square foot), seven-stage building (7). We defined a 'simulation hospital' (Figure 28.3) as a replica of a real full hospital environment where various types of healthcare workers can be trained in an immersive, multidisciplinary and longitudinal fashion throughout the continuum of the patient's pathway.

Conclusion

Simulation in a medical city such as the one at CRESENT is challenging and complex. Ensuring immersive environments, multidisciplinary education, longitudinal training and delivering of non-clinical simulation have all been key to the successful establishment of the simulation programme. Furthermore, system integration and patient experience simulation are innovative ways to develop the use of simulation in a medical city.

References

Kim, S., Hewitt, W., Buis, J. and Ross, B.K. (2015) Creating the infrastructure for a successful simulation program, in *Defining excellence in simulation programs* (eds J.C. Palaganas, J.C. Maxworthy, C.A. Epps and M.E. Mancini), Wolters Kluwer, Philadelphia, PA, pp. 66–89.

Lababidi, H. and Munshi, F. (2015) Development of simulation curriculum in postgraduate programs. *J Health Spec*, **3** (1), 17–21.

Joint Commission Resources. *The Joint Commission guide to improving staff communication*, 2nd ed. Oakbrook Terrace, IL: Joint Commission Resources; 2009.

ANZCA. Guidelines for transport of critically ill patients [cited 16 September 2016]. Available at: http://www.anzca.edu.au/documents/ps52-2015-guidelines-for-transport-of-critically-i.pdf

Frengley, R., Weller, J., Fanzca, M. *et al.* (2011) The effect of a simulation-based training intervention on the performance of established critical care unit teams. *Crit Care Med*, **39** (12), 2605–11.

Kobayashi, L., Shapiro, M.J., Sucov, A. *et al.* (2006) Portable advanced medical simulation for new emergency department testing and orientation. *Acad Emerg Med*, **13** (6), 691–5.

Lababidi, H., Munshi, F., AlAmar, M. *et al.* (2015) CRESENT: The Center for Research, Education and Simulation Enhanced Training, King Fahad Medical City, Riyadh. *Saudi Arabia. J Surg Simul.*, **2**, 42–6.

CHAPTER 29

'Who' and 'how' in simulation centre development: Buddies and ground rules

Eric So, George Ng & LY Ho

> **KEY MESSAGES**
>
> - Identification of internal and external partners early in simulation centre development is essential.
> - A clear governance and centre management structure is necessary before the simulation centre can go to the next stage of aligning its mission and vision to staff training needs and available resources.

Overview

This chapter summarizes the setting up of a Multidisciplinary Simulation and Skills Centre (MDSSC) in an acute public tertiary referral regional hospital, the Queen Elizabeth Hospital (QEH) in Hong Kong, China. We describe how the support of senior executives from the parent hospital and Hospital Authority (HA) of Hong Kong, commitment by a group of trainers passionate about simulation training and input from international simulation experts formed the foundation for subsequent development. We also discuss the steps the MDSSC has taken for continuous centre quality improvement and providing a high standard of healthcare through simulation training since it opened in 2011.

What was the need?

Contemporary medicine is complex, effective but potentially dangerous [1]. The Multidisciplinary Simulation and Skills Centre (MDSSC) is co-located within a hospital that provides elective and emergency inpatient services for most medical and surgical health issues across the lifespan. The MDSSC was set up in response to challenges in manpower and training, and aims to provide a safe learning environment for both trainers and participants. Expert clinicians, as advanced learners, need rehearsal of new procedures or complex situations where ideal team work is the central aim. Trainees, as beginning clinicians, need more focus on the deliberate practice of routine technical procedures before these are performed on real patients [2]. In addition, communication problems account for 70% of error in medicine [3], there is an obvious need for individual and team training on these critical, so called non-technical skills, contextualized within all levels of simulation training. The goal of the centre is to provide effective and efficient training for healthcare practitioners of different levels of experience on a range of skill sets through facility-based simulation and in-situ simulation. In this way, the capacity and competence of the healthcare workforce can be strengthened, with the aim of better patient safety and quality care.

What did we do?

Matching resources to needs

The MDSSC evolved as a result of needs from several areas. The senior hospital management through strategic planning recognized the training needs of the workforce, and the different clinical departments requested specialism-specific training to align with the requirements of the Hospital Authority (HA, a statutory body in Hong Kong managing all public hospitals and

---

Healthcare Simulation Education: Evidence, Theory and Practice, First Edition.
Edited by Debra Nestel, Michelle Kelly, Brian Jolly and Marcus Watson.
© 2018 John Wiley & Sons Ltd. Published 2018 by John Wiley & Sons Ltd.

institutes). Clinicians involved in the planning phase were convinced that simulation was a powerful and effective educational strategy when used strategically. Initial funding for the project came from charity donations and the hospital. It took almost two years from initial planning to the final opening of the centre.

The MDSSC was set up in a 650 square metre area originally used as an operating theatre. Most of the initial effort was spent on the environmental design of the centre, audio-visual technical infrastructure and control facilities, centre manpower requirements and clarity around staff roles and responsibilities. The environmental design concentrated on the realism of simulation training spaces according to likely scenarios, facility space distribution for various types of training, working spaces for the administrative team and storage areas for equipment [4].

As a novice team, we learnt from other well-established simulation centres locally and internationally to understand the basic principles of design and function. Fortunately, the steering committee (SC) was set up very early to provide focus and advice for centre development. The SC was the governance structure and comprised the hospital chief executive, hospital general managers, quality and safety director, major clinical department heads and the MDSSC directors and manager. The SC analysed hospital training needs to match the functional requirements of the centre within the constraints of the budget and facility space design. In the context of the multiple specialisms at the Queen Elizabeth Hospital (QEH), as well as the vision and mission of the hospital, the centre was designed for multidisciplinary cross-specialism simulation and skills training. In the original floor plan layout, there was a simulated operating room, an endovascular simulation and skills lab, a multifunction lecture room, a wet lab and control and debriefing rooms. A resuscitation room was added in 2015. The centre layout was designed for team-based scenario simulations, debriefing, skills stations, lectures and practice on animal specimens.

Its design was a balance of efficiency and flexibility in the use of existing spaces and the cost of replicating the hospital's clinical environment to maximize realism, while adhering to accepted architectural and educational concepts and theories. The ultimate purpose of the centre design was to engage learners in an immersive and reflective experience [5, 6].

Prioritization of goals

The MDSSC opened its doors in April 2011 and was lucky to receive adequate resources from the outset to support fiscal, human and material needs. The next step was to set early, realistic goals that could be accomplished to avoid overly ambitious targets. The MDSSC had to decide what the priority for investment was. The SC had the belief that committed staff were more important than expensive equipment. Apart from one high-tech mannequin simulator, the audio-visual system and a couple of donated task trainers, other centre equipment was inexpensive.

The MDSSC was started by doctors with proficient clinical knowledge, but who were less familiar with the concepts of adult learning, educational psychology, organizational behaviour and centre management. Issenberg [7] illustrated that the effectiveness of a simulation training programme was determined by the presence of three components: the training resources, trained educators and curricular institutionalization. The quality of the simulation educators and integration of simulation-based medical education (SBME) into the hospital's culture and mission were the top priorities for our early development. After careful discussion, we chose investment in educator training.

Intensive faculty development

The first formal training class for centre-based simulation educators was organized one month after the MDSSC officially opened. Experts from renowned international simulation centres were invited to the MDSSC to run a certified three-day training course. Many experienced front-line hospital clinicians and nurses from different departments applied. Selection of participants went through a stringent process, with review of applicants' teaching experience and curriculum vitae, since the number of applicants was overwhelming. Simulation training was very resource intensive and we wanted to select the right people. Successful applicants needed to make a commitment to future teaching in the MDSSC before they were formally accepted. Those who were accepted were drawn from different surgical and medical specialisms. The quality and safety department senior manager was also invited to join as the first step of our wider collaboration.

The train-the-trainer course provided participants with an adequate understanding of SBME. By the end, we had successfully cultivated and nurtured participants as champions. Shortly after the course, these champions from different departments started to develop their own interprofessional training courses for doctors and specialist nurses, such as a postpartum haemorrhage workshop (obstetricians) and an obstetric emergencies workshop for the emergency department (ED physicians, obstetricians and paediatricians).

We have already run five formal simulation train-the-trainer courses with a total of 115 credentialled simulation instructors according to the HA Standards. These instructors provide an important manpower resource for the HA and hospital-developed courses that run in the MDSSC. Some champions are also passionate about developing an interprofessional simulation training course as a new project for the hospital and the HA, which have already been rolled out or are in the development phase. It is the innovation, enthusiasm, grit and hard work of these champions that have helped the MDSSC to establish a track record of delivering high-quality simulation training courses, and to obtain buy-in from stakeholders and credibility within and external to the facility. These trained instructors and champions are no doubt the most valuable intangible assets of the centre (Figure 29.1). The MDSSC understands the importance of continuous faculty development in upholding training standards. Advanced trainer courses and refresher programmes have been arranged from time to time to fuel the instructors' intrinsic motivation.

Integration into the hospital

The SC is an important component and a convenient way for the MDSSC to maintain a connection between its activity and the hospital's strategic goals and initiatives. Through the SC, the MDSSC can simultaneously meet the needs of QEH and remain flexible to adapt to the organization's changing educational needs. Aligning the centre's training with the hospital's activities is important, since it ensures that the innovation of simulation training is recognized and permeates to different units and to all staff, and that contemporary practice contributes to the focus of the scenarios. In this way, it can be widely adopted as early as possible, because people see the value of the education modality through training partners within clinical departments. By listening to stakeholders, from top hospital management to individual participants, the MDSSC can take note of the perspectives of the different key stakeholders. This type

of dialogue helps the MDSSC to review its direction, its role in hospital operations and its strategic planning in developing and delivering educational programmes. It is also an important means of building trust and confidence among the hospital administration, clinical departments, instructors, participants and the centre. This mutual understanding offers the best opportunity for improving patient safety and achieving the centre's mission.

Accreditation process

When the MDSSC moved from a novice state to a more mature state, it started to evaluate how it could develop in a healthy direction. In 2012, it decided to enrol in a centre accreditation programme to provide quality healthcare education and to gain recognition for creative education. In preparation, the ADDIE (analysis, design, development, implementation and evaluation) education model [8] was incorporated into a curriculum proposal form for standardization of processes and the Curriculum Committee was set up. The Curriculum Committee was formed by a panel of experienced simulation instructors to vet submitted course proposals, to provide feedback and to offer recommendations for modification in the curriculum development process. This is to ensure that simulation is used within a systems-based approach as part of a wider curriculum. The MDSSC also noticed that clear centre policies and procedures were also very useful in filtering requests and prioritizing service provision according to the training curriculum structure and target participants in the sea of an overwhelming number of service requests. These policies and procedures were also essential to ensure the achievement of defined standards and educational quality improvement, which formed a crucial part of centre accreditation.

After more than a year of preparation and hard work by the centre administrative and technical team, the MDSSC was successfully accredited by the Society of Simulation in Healthcare on the training/education standard in May 2014 [9].

What was the impact?

Although infrastructure and personnel shape the MDSSC, it is its activities and the work it does that defines it. Developing and collecting metrics that accu-

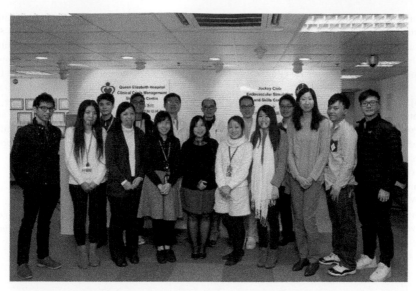

Figure 29.1 MDSSC department photo with the administrative, simulation and IT team members. Centre directors in second row: Dr LY Ho (third from left), Dr Eric So (third from right), Dr George Ng (second from right).

rately and consistently describe the activities of the simulation centre are mandatory. It will be useful when the MDSSC plans and projects future activities.

In the past few years, the number and breadth of learners have grown dramatically and the simulation courses have been typically well received by participants and faculty alike. The MDSSC runs recurrent HA courses (Intern Boot Camp Training, ECMO Simulation Training, Central Intern Orientation, CRM Scenario-Based Training) and hospital courses (Medication Safety Scenario Training, Transport of Critically Ill Patient Training, Ventilatory Support for Critically Ill Patient Training, Recovery Room Training Course) [10]. The allocation of training sessions is hospital programmes (80%), HA programmes (15%) and others (5%). Simulation-based and skill-based training participant numbers and contact hours in the MDSSC increased from 3170 participants and 10,800 hours in 2012 to 4120 participants and 23,300 hours in 2014, respectively.

Other performance indicators include learners' and facilitators' post-course evaluations and comments. Analysis of these provides useful information to enhance both participants' and instructors' learning and teaching and the viability of centre operations.

Taking into consideration the continuously evolving hospital organizational culture and context, the MDSSC will regularly evaluate its mission, vision and operational priorities through strategic planning with stakeholders. The centre will continue to work locally and think globally in its consistent, planned and collaborative application of SBME to ensure sustainability and contemporary offerings.

What lessons were learnt?

- Establish the governance and organizational framework of the centre at an early stage.
- Develop a service plan, a management plan and a budget plan to guide the centre's direction and daily operations.
- No simulation centre can work in isolation. It has to build passionate commitment, create champions and nurture advocates to achieve its mission through a shared purpose, shared ownership and a shared vision.

References

1 Chantler, C. (1999) The role and education of doctors in the delivery of healthcare. *Lancet*, **353**, 1178–81.

2 Crochet, P., Aggarwal, R., Dubb, S.S. *et al.* (2011) Deliberate practice on a virtual reality laparoscopic simulator enhances the quality of surgical technical skill. *Ann Surg*, **253** (6), 1216–22.

3 Joint Commission on Accreditation of Healthcare Organizations. 2016 National Patient Safety Goals [cited 16 September 2016]. Available at: www.jointcommission.org/PatientSafety/NationalPatientSafetyGoals/

4 Bradley, P. and Postlethwaite, K. (2003) Setting up a clinical skills learning facility. *Med Educ*, **37** (1), 6–13.

5 Rudolph, J.W., Simon, R. and Raemer, D.B. (2007) Which reality matters? Questions on the road to high engagement in healthcare simulation. *Simul Healthc*, **2** (3), 161–3.

6 Dieckmann, P., Manser, T., Wehner, T. and Rall, M. (2007) Reality and fiction cues in medical patient simulation: an interview study with anesthesiologists. *J Cogn Eng Decis Mak*, **1** (2), 148–68.

7 Issenberg, S.B. (2006) The scope of simulation-based healthcare education. *Simul Healthc*, **1** (4), 203–8.

8 Dick, W., Carey, L. and Carey, J.O. (2011) *The systematic design of instruction*, 7th edn, Pearson, Boston, MA.

9 Society for Simulation in Healthcare. SSH accreditation of healthcare simulation programs [cited 16 September 2016]. Available at: www.ssih.org/Accreditation

10 MDSSC. Multidisciplinary Simulation and Skills Centre [cited 16 September 2016]. Available at: http://www3.ha.org.hk/qeh/department/mdssc/en&uscore;index.html

Further Reading

1 Jeffries, P. and Battin, J. (2012) *Developing successful health care education simulation centers: the consortium model*, Springer, New York.

CHAPTER 30

Operationalizing a new emergency department: The role of simulation

Mike Eddie, Carrie Hamilton, Owen Hammett, Phil Hyde, Kate Pryde & Kim Sykes

KEY MESSAGES

- Large-scale environmental simulation demonstrates structural, functional and staffing challenges within proposed new builds; addressing these during the planning stage improves patient experience and saves money.

- Involvement of staff, simulated patients and simulated relatives/carers reinforces ownership.

- Overestimation of quantity of faculty and breadth of communication with stakeholders is essential.

Overview

Computer simulation models are frequently employed in the design of environmental spaces in both healthcare and industry [1, 2]. This approach employs complex software to enact a conceptual model of the environment of interest. Users of the system are third parties in such 'simulation' events. We describe the engagement of front-line staff and simulated patients in a large-scale simulation of a new children's emergency department (CED) prior to its internal fit-out.

What was the need?

As part of the development of a new children's hospital, it was proposed that the children's area within the existing emergency department (ED) amalgamate with the children's assessment unit (a ward-based general practitioner referral unit) to form a single children's emergency department (CED). Evidence from industry

suggests that environmental simulation can facilitate effective redesign and cost savings [3]. We planned a large-scale in-situ simulation to assess the functionality of the proposed CED prior to the internal fit-out. The simulation aimed to identify the impact of physical structure and staffing levels on patient care and experience, departmental efficiency and safety. We wanted the lessons learnt from the simulation to inform the design of the final build.

What did we do?

The architect's plans were taken to the construction company, the facilities department and hospital managers, who agreed to construct a temporary model of the proposed CED within the new hospital shell. The contractors built firewalls and made access points and stairwells safe for the simulation. Temporary flooring, heating and walls were installed, separating the shell into the areas defined on the architect's plan, for example majors (acute) and minors (sub-acute) areas, X-ray department, offices and so on. Each area was equipped to resemble a functioning ED. An information technology (IT) and telephone system was installed enabling patient 'notes' to be created and tests to be requested in real time. This allowed accurate tracking of each patient's pathway through the department.

We reviewed attendance patterns to the existing ED to generate the patient case mix of a typical shift. Fifty-three patient scenarios were created, ranging from minor injuries and illness to major 'code-blue' trauma. Every scenario included a storyboard for both

Healthcare Simulation Education: Evidence, Theory and Practice, First Edition.
Edited by Debra Nestel, Michelle Kelly, Brian Jolly and Marcus Watson.
© 2018 John Wiley & Sons Ltd. Published 2018 by John Wiley & Sons Ltd.

the simulated patient (SP) and the accompanying simulated parent/carer, including information on mode of arrival – walking, ambulance; props required – buggies, wheelchairs, siblings, elderly relatives; physical and psychological aspects of the case; and the expected progress of the scenario. A timeline was constructed detailing when each SP would arrive in the department. The SPs and their parents/carers were sourced from our organization's SP programme. We held a pre-event training day for the SPs and faculty to outline the aims and context of the exercise, as well as logistics for the day including a safety briefing. Individual storyboards were reviewed with the SPs by a member of the faculty and additional information to aid accurate depiction of the role added as required. Access to support from the SP team for the participants was available at all stages of the process. Consent for the entire event, including debriefing, was gained from everyone.

The simulation took place on a Saturday to minimize impact on service provision and to facilitate access to equipment. The area was prepared in the preceding days by the faculty and undergraduate healthcare students from the critical care programme (CCP). Representatives from management, facilities and contracting (subject experts) were positioned and tasked with providing focused feedback. Each area had two to three simulation faculty members to facilitate the scenarios and support the SPs. Faculty and subject experts wore different-coloured T-shirts to identify them as non-participants. The event was audio-visually (AV) recorded by a roaming film crew for review in the feedback phase.

On the day of the simulation, staff arrived in uniform and undertook a safety briefing and tour of the site. They were then positioned in their working areas. The staffing mix included paramedics, administrative staff, nurses, doctors, radiographers, plaster technicians and play therapists, reflecting the proposed staffing model of the new department. Additional specialist medical staff were available if requested. The simulation was designed to incorporate handover from day to night teams and required two shifts of staff. Staff took breaks as per a normal shift and refreshments were provided.

The SPs were accommodated in a separate area. As each SP entered the simulation, they were provided with an age-appropriate feedback form. Feedback was structured to capture their experience as a patient in the new department and as a participant in the simulation.

A number of SPs were positioned in the scenario at the start. Staff familiarized themselves with the SPs and a claxon sounded to start the event. Subsequent SPs joined the simulation according to the pre-determined timeline, each escorted by a CCP student. SPs arriving by ambulance entered the spaces on trolleys accompanied by a paramedic and went straight to the resuscitation room if necessary. Staff assessed, instigated laboratory and/or diagnostic investigations and treated SPs in real time. SPs were taken to 'X-ray', medication was prepared in the 'drug preparation area' and bloods were taken by porters to the 'lab'. SPs were either admitted or discharged, at which point they were escorted back to the SP preparation area and debriefed.

Multisource feedback was captured throughout the simulation from subject experts, SPs, staff and faculty. SPs and simulated relatives/carers had paper feedback forms and interactive maps on which to record their journey. The temporary walls functioned as white boards and staff were able to write feedback/observations on these during the simulation. All staff involved attended an immediate 'hot' debrief facilitated by the simulation faculty. This captured instant reaction and immediate concerns about their experience in the simulation. They were given a paper feedback form to complete, which was emailed again the following week, giving them a further opportunity to reflect and feedback. Over the next three months, feedback was presented at discussion sessions with all stakeholders to enable utilization of the data in the redesign process.

What was the impact?

Patient flow through the simulated department demonstrated clear structural, functional and staffing challenges within the proposed design. There was no dedicated resuscitation area in the new design. A child requiring resuscitation needed to be transferred through the waiting room to the combined resuscitation room in the main ED. Paediatric-trained staff had to accompany the patient, compromising flow in the CED due to a reduction in staff numbers. The alternative was to manage resuscitation alongside less acute patients.

There was no area available to triage patients when they arrived in the majors (acute) area. The cubicles were isolated from the rest of the clinical activity and although there was a dedicated staff workstation, it was no more than a shelf attached to a wall in a corridor. It had no visual communication with other areas in the department. The lack of a waiting/changing area for X-ray (located next to the CED entrance) meant that patients were waiting in a main thoroughfare. The location of the staff workstations was sub-optimal for a number of reasons, including being adjacent to play areas (which compromised confidentiality) and having no line of sight to the beds where the sickest patients were located. The drug preparation room had a large pillar in the centre that rendered the floor space unusable. The play area contained a clinical sink, which was a potential hazard.

The feedback enabled the interior of the new department to be redesigned to address these issues. If we had not recognized these problems until after the department had been built, it would have cost in excess of £50,000 to rectify. If the layout had been constructed as proposed, it would have necessitated three extra staff per shift (compared to prior modelling) in order to run the department safely. Three extra staff would incur an annual cost of £100,000 or £2 million over the lifetime of the department (20 years).

Involvement of a wide range of hospital staff, SPs and simulated parents/carers meant that all felt engaged in the design of their local service. Traditionally, staff and patients only have the opportunity to feedback on new designs based on information shared electronically or on paper. Actually 'working' in the simulated department allowed for a level of feedback from staff that would not normally be captured in a consultation exercise. For the SPs, parents and carers, this exercise allowed them to co-design a system at the outset based on their simulated experience. For the faculty, it allowed us to develop expertise in large-scale simulation, on which we are now able to provide advice and practical help to other departments and institutions.

What lessons were learnt?

A successful large-scale simulation requires a sizeable, experienced faculty. For us, access to a multidisciplinary group of undergraduate healthcare students (CCP)

was invaluable in maintaining the flow of participants throughout the day. It was a unique opportunity for them as prospective healthcare providers. Individual responsibility for the organization of the components of the event needs to be very clear. Widely advertising the simulation throughout the organization allows stakeholders to raise concerns before the event and minimizes unanticipated reactions on the day.

Having a detailed faculty 'walk-through' of the arrival of SPs into the simulation enables them to predict how many high-acuity scenarios may be running simultaneously. This helps to target the number of faculty needed in each area. Staff taking part in the exercise need more preparation and familiarization than one might anticipate. Many staff have experienced simulation as part of their training and continuing professional development, but most have not participated in anything on this scale. It should be anticipated that some people will feel that they are going to be judged on their individual performance and become stressed. One strategy to reduce this occurring is to have a good amount of time at the start of the event to allow familiarization with the environment and the SPs already positioned in the simulation. We could also have introduced pauses into the simulation to allow staff to clarify any concerns they had about the simulated environment.

Conclusion

This exercise demonstrated that the design of complex systems can be achieved using large-scale, multimodal, in-situ simulation. The feedback catalysed a redesign of the internal space, a rethinking of patient flow and a reorganization of staff utilization within the proposed CED. Simulated child patients and their parents/carers brought the clinical space to life, drawing staff into the simulation and providing the child's perspective on issues such as confidentiality and aesthetics. It generated feedback that could not be obtained from paper/computer modelling. The simulation provided the opportunity for changes to be implemented prior to building the actual department, preventing the exposure of real patients to the safety, staffing and environmental threats posed by the original design and saving an estimated £2 million. This simulation project demonstrated how staff, children and families can contribute meaningfully to the design of clinical spaces within healthcare.

References

1 Gunal, M.M. (2012) A guide for building hospital simulation models. *Healthc Syst.*, **1**, 17–25.
2 The Cumberland Initiative. Leading NHS figures urge health service to use computer modelling to resolve winter A+E Crisis [cited 16 September 2016]. Available at: http://www.cumberland-initiative.org/2013/07/21/fixing-emergency-care/
3 HSJ. Take urgent care for a test drive [cited 16 September 2016]. Available at: http://www.hsj.co.uk/home/innovation-and-efficiency/take-urgent-care-for-a-test-drive/5066922.article

CHAPTER 31

Simulation modelling and analysis to test health systems

Kenny Macleod & Robert Moody

KEY MESSAGES

- Health systems can be complex and difficult to get right first time, but there are tools to reduce the risk of getting it wrong.

- Simulation allows designers and managers to learn about how their plans will work, prior to the proposed build or change.

- Simulation modelling identifies the most cost-effective and efficient options for processes, layouts, capacities and resource balance.

Overview

Healthcare systems comprise a complex mix of resources and processes, with resources often being stretched, resulting in delays in care. Simulation modelling of health systems allows stakeholders to learn about their environment and try out small or even major changes to see if they can make improvements, without having an impact on patients.

This simple case study shows how simulation modelling helped design a breast-screening facility. Layouts, processes, staffing and resources were all included in the model to determine how they might work together in the most efficient manner.

The learning is twofold: as well as simulation being used as a tool to improve layout and processes, it can also be used as a management training tool, in the same way as physical, medical simulators support skills and team work.

What was the need?

Screening for breast cancer is a high priority on the Australian healthcare agenda [1]. Breast cancer screening, the examination of people with no symptoms, is a common preventative strategy for early detection in those with unsuspected disease. Mammography is the key imaging modality in breast cancer diagnosis. BreastScreen Victoria is a state-based organization and part of BreastScreen Australia, the national population-screening programme for women. This programme, free of charge to all eligible women, was designed to detect breast cancer at an early stage, when treatment is most likely to be successful.

Demand for breast cancer screening is increasing. BreastScreen Victoria currently screens 60% of its target demographic (women 50–69 years of age) [2]. The national standard is that the programme should screen 70% of this group [3]. One site that offers the screening programme is St Vincent's Hospital (Melbourne), a large inner-city tertiary public healthcare service. The hospital's breast screening catchment area encompasses southeastern and northern metropolitan areas of Melbourne and the rural Victorian area of Goulburn Valley. The creation of increased screening capability for the inner-city catchment is required to allow for this projected growth in demand.

To meet the demand, a new breast cancer screening clinic, the Rose Clinic, was to be established within a city-based department store (David Jones). The aim of this new service was to offer women a more inviting environment that was convenient and less intimidating

Healthcare Simulation Education: Evidence, Theory and Practice, First Edition.
Edited by Debra Nestel, Michelle Kelly, Brian Jolly and Marcus Watson.
© 2018 John Wiley & Sons Ltd. Published 2018 by John Wiley & Sons Ltd.

compared with hospital-based facilities. The planned throughput of the new facility was projected as between 6000 and 12,000 mammography screens per annum. Although the clinic will have the capacity for two full field digital mammography units, the throughput is based on only one unit being utilized.

FlexSim computer simulation software, supported locally by TMN Simulation (www.tmn.com.au), was chosen to assist with designing the Rose Clinic to deliver the best patient experience.

Purpose

- Assist St Vincent's Hospital Melbourne and BreastScreen Victoria's planning and operational teams with developing a suitable clinic layout.
- Inform the David Jones department store's planning, design and building teams of the requirements for a suitable facility plan for partner approval and subsequent specification for the construction of a suitable clinic.
- Identify resources required for the predicted throughput, for example the number of scanners, changing rooms, seating and staffing.

What was included

Clinic floor plan design:
- Consideration of patient workflow
- Consideration of modalities (scanner) to be used and related equipment
- Consideration of office equipment to support clinic administration
- Consideration of relevant healthcare facilities, codes and standards

Constraints

- The size of the available floor space suitable for the intended use
- Phased deployment of mammography modality

Why the simulation was considered

The establishment of a new healthcare clinic allowed for the review of processes and the consideration of best practices in the design of the new facility, and simulation modelling is the only viable option to measure and visualize something that does not already exist.

The alternative is to use expert opinion or replicate an existing facility, neither of which could prove that the new facility would run efficiently.

In particular, establishing this clinic had additional considerations:
- It was located in a non-clinical setting
- It allowed the introduction of new digital diagnostic/imaging modalities

What did we do?

As healthcare processes are often complex and difficult to convey clearly, it was felt that a simulation tool would help in stakeholder communications by ensuring a more complete understanding of the processes and interactions involved. Presenting a three-dimensional (3D) visualization, backed with observed data (that is, a model that both looks and acts like the proposed solution) is a very visual approach and tells a compelling story to encourage stakeholder understanding and buy-in.

Using the simulation

Healthcare computer simulation was used to assist with the design and understanding of the overall process for the new Rose Clinic.

The functionality of the chosen application, FlexSim Healthcare HC, aligned well with project requirements. FlexSim HC is a 3D, virtual reality, simulation application based on patient pathways: it helps with visualizing physical layout and process designs.

A patient pathway (aka patient track or experience) is a structured sequence of events; activity timings; staff and resource requirements; locations; problems; and decisions that a patient will experience during their visit. With the specialist nature of this facility, only one patient pathway was developed.

The software was used to model a number of scenarios:
- The use of one X-ray machine vs two machines
- The use of changing rooms vs changing in the mammography room
- The use of one changing room vs two changing rooms
- The use of one radiographer vs two radiographers for two modalities
- The entire clinic layout design
- The time taken to do each task, such as registration, changing and breast screen

To start, an empty floorplan was laid out in the simulated clinic. The objects that represented the equipment, staff and patients were then added to the model.

Building on the base model, the scenarios were developed using the experimenter function, which allows the model to be run through multiple replications. Alternative scenario development involved such things as the grouping of radiographers, repositioning their home base, adding new paths between the mammography rooms, greater throughput of patients and altering the number of changing rooms. Different layouts were investigated by moving the objects into new areas.

The FlexSim application allowed for running and verification of the object interactions within each scenario. Dynamic animations and charts were displayed onscreen and output as an AVI video file. Performance data were exported for further analysis.

What was the impact?

The healthcare simulation modelling software allowed for the examination of and experimentation with various scenario outcomes that supported informed decision making for the Rose Clinic design. Based on the positive experience of this project, simulation modelling was used by the St Vincent's Hospital Project Management Office team to assist with patient flows for a new heart centre, and is currently assisting with the development of service models for a planned $120 million ambulatory and integrated care centre. Although in its infancy within the health industry, the use of simulation modelling will benefit healthcare providers through a greater understanding of facility flows and utilization. This will lead to improved workflows; reduced inefficiencies and costs; and increased staff and patient satisfaction. It is therefore highly likely that simulation software will become an essential part of future clinical redesign and a tool for future project teams.

What lessons were learnt?

The healthcare simulation allowed for the examination of various scenario outcomes that supported informed decision making for the 'Rose Clinic' design. The main area of focus was how to structure the changing rooms to allow for an efficient throughput of patients, with a secondary focus on patient flow and the capacity of the waiting room.

There were two main lessons to be learnt from this exercise:

- From a numerical and logical point of view, simulation modelling demonstrated and confirmed the most efficient ways to carry out the tasks.
- Altering and comparing alternative simulation scenarios supports decision makers in selecting which option best fits their decision criteria. This can be capital decisions, such as one diagnostic machine or two, or operational decisions relating to, say, staffing and procedures.

By a process of comparing and experimenting, the number of changing rooms were considered (one, two and no changing rooms). The outcome was that two parallel changing rooms were proven to be the most efficient use of the radiographer's time and improved overall procedural times. Specifically, the use of two changing rooms allowed adequate patient privacy; one patient could get ready for the scan while the other was getting dressed to leave.

Next steps

While noting social and qualitative issues, healthcare simulation modelling and analysis will be extended to ensure the best possible patient experience and workflow efficiency in areas such as:

- care pathways
- patient flow
- maximizing use of equipment and facilities
- staffing levels and utilization
- streamlining admissions and patient care processes
- facility planning

Simulation modelling and analysis tools specifically designed to model care pathways are relatively new to healthcare; but there is also benefit in drawing experience from other industries where simulation modelling is a mature technology. Customer (patient) support and throughput, supply chain and logistics, call centres, building design, resource balancing, scheduling and so on are all areas in common with other industries.

Initially, simulation modelling in healthcare would be most useful in supporting business cases, planning, resourcing and process improvement. The biggest

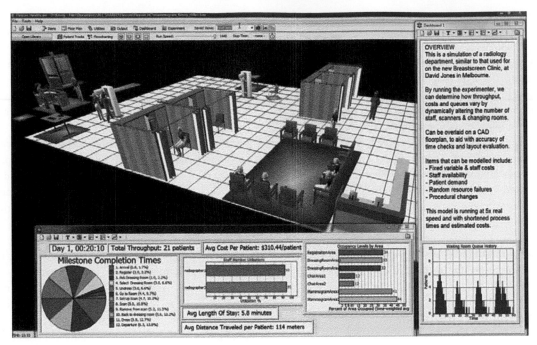

Figure 31.1 The simulation running with two X-ray machines, each having two changing areas. The metrics displayed include census, costs, throughput, completion times, length of stay, distance walked and so on.

applicability and impact are likely to be realized in these areas within healthcare. Over time, standard models may be built up that will form the basis for the development of future scenarios. This will speed up and simplify the development process and lead to the further use of simulation modelling, that in time will be of wider benefit to the healthcare industry.

What the simulation did to benefit the project

Like other simulation activities outlined in this book, this project provided a synthetic but realistic environment. The software created much interest within the project and redesign teams, and there were sufficient 3D realism and metrics to give stakeholders confidence that decisions being made on the different scenarios of layouts, capacity and resources were the best choices.

The 3D models created (Figure 31.1) certainly looked impressive and the benefits of using FlexSim HC were readily apparent on viewing its capabilities.

The scenarios aided in the communication design processes and allowed for discussions regarding planned and future usage of the clinic. This is because the model made it easy to view the various layout plans and comprehend the implications of various processes and interactions on functions and business.

Simulation modelling and analysis were very useful as tools to assist with understanding the design considerations for the planning of the Rose Clinic. The simulation software, FlexSim HC, supported the experience of the clinicians and consultant practitioners, who are well versed on the design requirements of the facility.

FlexSim HC is a useful tool that will increasingly be called on in the future to maximize decision effectiveness for process design. The relative ease with which scenarios may be examined means that it will be a factor not only in the planning phase, but also after the launch of the clinic.

References

1 Australian Institute of Health and Welfare. National health priority areas [cited 25 November 2015]. Available at: http://www.aihw.gov.au/national-health-priority-areas/

2 BreastScreen Victoria. Health professionals [cited 17 October 2015]. Available at https://www.breastscreen.org.au/Professionals

3 BreastScreen Australia. Background [cited 20 November 2015]. Available at: https://www.bcna.org.au/about-us/advocacy/position-statements/breastscreen-australia/

4 Gartner. Gartner identifies the top 10 strategic technology trends for 2013 [cited 15 October 2015]. Available at: http://www.gartner.com/newsroom/id/2209615

Further Reading

1 Macleod K. Design of layout and process of the Rose Clinic. *A breast-screen facility facilitated by St Vincent's Hospital Melbourne*. Paper presented at SimTect 2014, Melbourne. Available at:https://www.researchgate.net/publication/281745653_Design_of_layout_and_process_of_the_Rose_Clinic._A_breast-screen_facility_facilitated_by_St_Vincent%27s_Hospital_Melbourne

2 TMN Simulation. David Jones breast screening facility [cited 16 September 2016]. Available at: https://youtu.be/lWTt8iI4-ao

Additional Resources

1 FlexSim simulation software, https://www.flexsim.com/textbook/

SECTION VI
Conclusions and future practice

SECTION VI

Conclusions and future practice

CHAPTER 32

Twenty years on ... forecasting healthcare simulation practices

Debra Nestel & Michelle Kelly

KEY MESSAGES

- Valuing patient safety will continue to be the principal driver for healthcare simulation practices.

- Professional associations will play an important role in advancing simulation practices by setting standards, certification of practitioners, refining and developing shared languages and more [1].

- Flexible funding models need to be established for future-proofing healthcare simulation.

- Healthcare consumers have an important role to play in shaping healthcare simulation practices.

Overview

This chapter considers the contents of this book with a view to forecasting educational practices in healthcare simulation. We return to the key issues of the role of simulation in patient safety and to the vision of Sir Liam Donaldson in 2007. We fast-forward 20 years and consider the contributions by section, addressing theoretical perspectives – whether they will be relevant; contemporary issues – whether they will be current; elements of simulation practice – whether they will be recognizable; and innovations in simulation – by definition there ought not to be any of those! It is an exciting future and hope that there is an opportunity to revisit this subject in 2037.

Introduction

The introduction to this book opened with the following quote:

> Simulation offers an important route to safer care for patients and needs to be more fully integrated into the health service.
> *Sir Liam Donaldson, 2009*

The contributions in this book demonstrate progress made towards addressing this vision. In our introduction we also indicated that we would finish the book by gazing into a crystal ball. We note the powerful message from Professor Harry Owen (Chapter 3) that for much of the twentieth century we have had to rediscover how simulation leads to safer healthcare practices. Even in the twenty-first century, we continue to work towards accumulating a body of evidence on the impact of simulation on the performance of healthcare students and professionals, and on the role of simulation in developing safer healthcare systems and practices.

Focusing on simulation as an educational method, we draw on the reflections of Regehr, who describes two dominant discourses in health professions education research and proposes that we reorientate them: from the imperative of proof to one of understanding; and from the imperative of simplicity to one of representing complexity well [2]. In 2016, on the launch of a new journal intended to provide a forum for advancing healthcare simulation, the editor-in-chief [DN] cited

---

Healthcare Simulation Education: Evidence, Theory and Practice, First Edition.
Edited by Debra Nestel, Michelle Kelly, Brian Jolly and Marcus Watson.
© 2018 John Wiley & Sons Ltd. Published 2018 by John Wiley & Sons Ltd.

this reorientation in publishing articles that seek understanding *with* and *about* simulation; how simulation leads to deeper learning, improved clinician performance and improved healthcare systems; and that simulation is well suited to explore, represent and discover the complexities of healthcare education, systems and care [3]. *Evidence* remains important, but other factors are likely to influence the uptake of simulation too. We acknowledge the impact of wider social, political, educational and economic trends.

Although it is exciting to forecast, a distant projection is probably less helpful than the near future. Many healthcare services seem to be designed with about a 20-year life before substantive redesign, so we will confine our projections to this time frame. We also acknowledge that entry-level health professional curricula are under constant review, with in our experience substantive changes made approximately every 10 years.

First, we return to Sections II to V of the book to inform our forecast. In Section II, we offered theories and frameworks to structure or order ways in which we might think about and practise using simulation. In the next 20 years we will see the advancement of theories and the emergence of new frameworks that better reflect our evolving practices. It is unlikely that there will ever be a unified theory of simulation; instead, theories of the middle range or practice-based theories will be posited, informing, challenging and extending our thinking and practices [4]. Theory will increasingly be conceptualized, adapted and applied to simulation, especially in the context of education [4]. The contested notion of realism will shift from focusing on achievement of the highest *fidelity* to being *fit for purpose* and offering *meaningfulness* for learners.

In Section III, Chapter 6 presents various published research strategies, priorities and questions relevant to simulation-based education (SBE), to surgery, to paediatrics and from a national perspective. These questions will continue to guide research and of course new ones will emerge. The remaining authors offered their perspectives on a range of contemporary issues, including human- and technology-based simulators and simulations. It is a privilege to have the opportunity to work in a field that can be informed by such diverse approaches as dramaturgy and haptics! Gaming will have greater prominence across all phases of health professions education. Three-dimensional printing in healthcare simulation will be commonplace. These

different approaches will continue to advance our field and others will enter it. We are likely to see concerted efforts to measure human performance through simulation and the use of performance data from clinical settings to inform simulation design. This section also included macro-level issues, including the role of simulation-specific professional associations – some of which are likely to grow, supporting members in different ways including regulation of practice, certification of members and credentialling of programmes. Although these exist in 2016, their uptake globally is limited. Simulation educators and operations specialists will be recognised for their expertise. Professional associations will ensure that simulation innovations are disseminated. Already the Society for Simulation in Healthcare is facilitating a global collaboration of simulation practitioners in developing a shared language [5].

The sustainability of healthcare simulation will continue to be discussed. New and flexible funding models will emerge, especially as simulation becomes embedded in curricula and certification in simulation for specific clinical tasks, specialist or advanced practices becomes mandatory. It will no longer be acceptable to use history as the basis for maintaining inefficient and outmoded training approaches. Importantly, the *political* positioning of the simulation director within the host institution will be at the executive level. The ability of simulation activities to *add value* to the healthcare service will be accepted (Chapter 15). We will see the criticality of simulation espoused at the highest levels, in much the same way that Donaldson emphasised its importance in 2007: specialist medical colleges, higher education institutions and healthcare services will have simulation leads and national patient safety agencies will work closely with simulation groups to enable learning from serious incidents. Levine et al. propose that healthcare education will become more regulated and therefore accountable and simulation will have a key role in this [6].

In Section IV, elements of simulation practice are shared. We will see shifts in some of these topics with the ethics of simulation, especially in education become a dominant discourse. Ethics and healthcare simulation already have a close and evolving relationship. This includes notions of deception, of caring for simulated participants and learners, of deriving scenarios from real clinical practice, of audio-visual recording, of incorporating training and assessment data in simulations.

Complex ethical issues in healthcare will be explored using simulation. Interprofessional and team-based healthcare is well established in many institutions and will become an even greater focus for SBE. Clinicians will come to expect to rehearse elements of clinical practice regularly in teams.

We will see refinement of the educational practices shared in Section IV. Even though simulation modalities are diverse, there appear to be commonalities in designing for learning using simulation. The NHET-Sim phases illustrate a systematic approach to simulation practice (Chapter 18), which appears in various chapters throughout the book. Over the next 20 years, this particular systematic approach will be challenged. We will also see the emergence of new simulation modalities. Chapter 21 is a superb collation of current issues in debriefing practices. In our field, debriefing has close to the status of a 'god term', in much the same way that Professor Lorelei Lingard describes the word 'competence' in medicine and education [7]. Debriefing has yielded a flourishing educational Industry with specific approaches shared internationally on fee-paying courses. Physical infrastructure has emerged to support debriefing practices. It would be hard to find a healthcare simulation conference that did not foreground debriefing. This holds benefits, including the careful examination of the technique, but there are also challenges if debriefing is privileged over deeper values and beliefs about simulation as an educational method. Much is written about debriefing, but there are still relatively few empirical studies. The next 20 years will see an orientation of debriefing embedded in the wider arc of SBE, valuing the importance and impact of thoughtful scenario design, of briefing, of promoting reflection, of assessment and of evaluation.

And in Section V, the innovations provide a feast of simulation practices from around the world. If in 20 years the opportunity arose to select a new set of innovations, then they may include examples of even greater integration of simulated participants with technology-based simulators, enabling realistic, complex and standardised approaches to support learning, performance and assessment. We may also have examples from continents not represented here, reflecting our own richer network. Simulation educators will be able to author scenarios in virtual worlds quickly and easily. They will share innovations associated with gaming. We may see examples of wearable technologies that

document clinicians' practices in simulation and also in clinical settings. Each will inform the other, especially in designing simulation activities that target elements of a clinician's work that require improvement. This data will also provide less experienced clinicians with exemplars of how to develop their practices. Of course, there will be examples of augmented reality combined with data feedback loops, again providing learners with information (just in time) to develop clinical skills and perhaps negating the presence of a clinical tutor. Technological advances in operative procedural techniques will always be underpinned by training in simulation.

We will see examples of cultural change in organizations that enable clinicians to have devoted practice times in the simulation centre or in-situ simulation. In the same way that a footballer practises skills or training drills that are found in every match and rehearses set plays with the team, so too will clinicians expect to use simulation to train for everyday situations, seeking always to refine their practice, to achieve excellence and to work optimally with others. Other innovations will include offering large cohorts of learners high-quality simulation-based curricula cognisant of the diversity, expectations and culturally contextual nature of learners [8]. We are also likely to see examples of seamless movement between learning in clinical and learning in simulated environments.

In this book we have only scratched the surface with respect to the applications of simulation in healthcare. A wider range of health and social care professions will be involved. Our focus has been on SBE for healthcare students and professionals, but the use of simulation to inform patients and their carers about health literacy, how to navigate the healthcare system and how to co-produce or engage more in self-management holds enormous potential. Healthcare consumers will routinely inform simulation practices.

Conclusion

The next 20 years are likely to be as exciting as the last two decades, in which there has been exponential growth in simulation education and research. The drivers are well documented and have largely been associated with patient safety, but the provision of training opportunities for large numbers of entry-level professionals and increasing accountability in clinicians' practice and educational quality are also important. Healthcare services and higher education providers must commit to supporting simulation. Access to simulation resources as an educational method has been patchy, but this is shifting, at least in many Western countries. There are still large parts of the world that have limited access to simulation. Of course, technology-based simulations may be constrained by local infrastructure, interest or commitment, but as we have seen in this book, much valuable simulation occurs without sophisticated technology. The model whereby clinicians personally pay for their own training makes little sense in healthcare services that truly place patients first. Simulation practitioners have a responsibility to lead elements of education and healthcare service reform. Perhaps the most exciting prospect is the maturation of the interdisciplinary nature of healthcare simulation and the inclusion of healthcare consumers to complement the development of holistic scenarios for students and clinicians. Although we look forward to 2037, we will make sure that we enjoy the journey with the contributors to this book and our many colleagues around the world.

References

1 Donaldson, L. (2009) 150 years of the Chief Medical Officer's Annual Report 2008, Department of Health, London.
2 Regehr, G. (2010) It's NOT rocket science: rethinking our metaphors for research in health professions education. *Med Educ.*, **44**, 31–9.
3 Nestel, D. (2016) Open access publishing in health and social care simulation research – Advances in Simulation. *Adv Simul.*, **1**, 2. doi: 10.1186/s41077-015-0002-x
4 Nestel, D. and Bearman, M. (2015) Theory and simulation-based education: definitions, worldviews and applications. *Clin Simul Nurs.*, **11**, 349–54.
5 Levine, A., DeMaria, S., Scwartz, A. and Sim, A. (2013) A future vision, in *The comprehensive textbook of healthcare simulation* (eds A. Levine, S. DeMaria, A. Schwartz and A. Sim), Springer, New York, pp. 649–54.
6 Lopreiato, J.O., Downing, D., Gammon, W., Lioce, L., Sittner, B., Slot, V., Spain, A.E. and the Terminology & Concepts Working Group (2016) Healthcare Simulation Dictionary. Retrieved from http://www.ssih.org/dictionary.
7 Lingard, L. (2009) What we see and don't see when we look at 'competence': Notes on a god term. *Adv Health Sci Educ*, **14** (5), 625–8.
8 Kelly, M.A., Hopwood, N., Rooney, D. and Boud, D. (2016) Enhancing students' learning through simulation: dealing with diverse, large cohorts. *Clin Simul Nurs*, **12** (5), 171–6.

Index

Healthcare Simulation Education: Evidence, Theory and Practice, First Edition.
Edited by Debra Nestel, Michelle Kelly, Brian Jolly and Marcus Watson.
© 2018 John Wiley & Sons Ltd. Published 2018 by John Wiley & Sons Ltd.

Printed and bound by CPI Group (UK) Ltd, Croydon, CR0 4YY

27/10/2024

14580194-0002